Get
STRONGER
by
STRETCHING
with Thera-Band®

Second Edition

D0745254

Get STRONGER by STRETCHING

with Thera-Band®

Second Edition

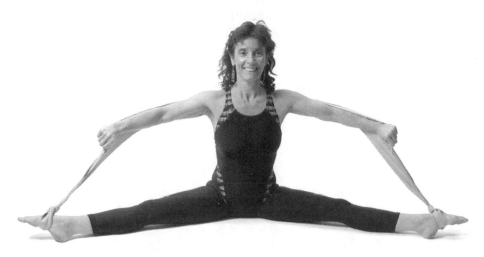

by Noa Spector-Flock

Princeton Book Company, Publishers
Hightstown, New Jersey

While every effort has been made to ensure that the content of this book is as technically accurate and as sound
as possible, neither the author, the Hygenic Corporation,
nor the publishers can accept responsibility for any injury
sustained as a result of the use of this material.

Readers are advised to consult a doctor prior to beginning
any exercise program.

Copyright ©2002 by Noa Spector-Flock.

All rights reserved. No part of this work may be reprinted
without the written permission of the author. Thera-Band®
is used with permission of the Hygenic Corporation.

Princeton Book Company, Publishers
P.O. Box 831
Hightstown, NJ 08520

Interior and cover design by Efrain Rivera, Jr.
Composition by Doric Lay Publishers

Library of Congress Cataloging-in-Publication Data

Spector-Flock, Noa.
    Get stronger by stretching with Thera-Band / by Noa Spector-
        Flock. — 2nd ed.
            p. cm.
    Includes bibliographical references.
    ISBN 0-87127-243-1 (pbk.)
        1. Stretching exercises. 2. Exercise. I. Title.

GV505 .S64 2002
613.7´1—dc21

                                                    2001058008

Printed in Canada
Second printing

Dedication

Dedication

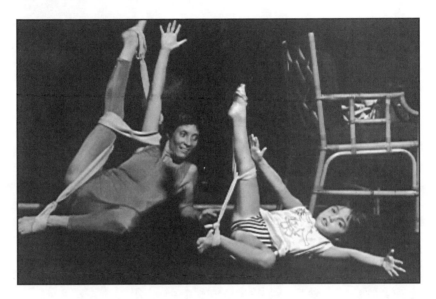

I was a bit nervous the first year that I taught at the University of South Florida in Tampa, Florida. My daughter Maya was between six months and one year old, so I would bring her along with me as I taught my class, Movement Awareness in the Spirit of Feldenkrais. At that time, she was learning to roll, sit, crawl, and stand up. She showed my class exactly what I was trying to teach them about simple, efficient, developmental movement. Maya actually did the teaching for me that year. It turned out to be one of my best years of teaching ever.

Thank you, Maya!

Table of Contents

Contents

Acknowledgments

Acknowledgments

1st edition

I would like to acknowledge the work of the following people who had patience with my English and contributed the time that was necessary to make this book come true: The Hygenic Corporation, the maker of the Thera-Band® products, which gave me the permission to use its product in my book; Don Musselman, who enriched my work with his wide knowledge of language, theater, and literature; my students who helped in the first stages of the creation: Alexandra Hahl, who edited, organized, and helped put the manuscript into good form; Peter Hahl, who provided the illustrations; Al Pritcher and Matt Johnson, who did the photography; Angela Rauter, Marlow Fleming, Michael, and David, who modeled for the exercises; and all my friends who were willing to read and give me their input and corrections.

Most important are the contributions of each and every one of my students in school and workshops, and clients young and old, from whom I have learned what I now share. All of you have made this book possible, and I thank you.

Noa Spector-Flock, 1991

2nd edition

I would like to acknowledge the work of the following people who helped in the preparation of the second edition of my book: The Hygenic Corporation, the maker of the Thera-Band® products, which gave me the permission to use its product in my book; Thera-Band® Academy; Phil Page, PT, ATC: Manager of Clinical Education and Research for Thera-Band®; Jennifer Baker of the American Physical Therapy Association (APTA); and Margaret Devenney of Trafford Publishing. Thank you to Paul Linden, Ph.D., for permission to adapt and use his drawings on pages 29 and 30. In addition, I must thank Bob Kowkabany of Doric Lay Publishers for making the book look so good. And I am most grateful to the staff at Princeton Book Company, Publishers, who worked so hard to design, edit, and publicize this book: Naomi Mindlin, editor; Deborah Blok, publicist; Efrain Rivera, Jr., graphic designer; and Lisa Denham, graphic designer. Finally, thank you to Charles Woodford, editor and owner of Princeton Book Company, without whom the second edition would not exist.

Again, my most important contributors remain my students and clients from whom I have learned what I continue to share. I thank you all very much.

Noa Spector-Flock, 2001

Preface
Preface

After World War II, there arose many new and varied approaches to the human body. This was especially true in physical education and modern dance. Growing up in Israel, I was fortunate to be exposed to many of these new approaches. I can remember watching my mother teach a class in yoga. Her students were people from all backgrounds—high school pupils, office workers who wanted to stretch, artists who were drawn to Eastern modes, dance teachers who were open to new ways of learning, as well as others. All were seated on the rug in our living room. The room had large windows, which had a beautiful view overlooking pine forests and the blue Mediterranean Sea. My mother's particular approach to yoga was based on her knowledge of astrology and on the changes of the months. She thought that by applying her knowledge of astrology with teaching yoga, her students would improve their physical health and mental well-being.

Several years later, when I was in school, I was subjected to a method of movement education that was very stiff and formal. My parents finally came to my rescue and sent me to ballet classes. This enabled me to enrich my movement vocabulary and, more important, to pursue my inner dreams.

In my desire for expression, I often spent my time at home dancing to old 78 RPM recordings of the Vienna Philharmonic playing Tchaikovsky's *Sleeping Beauty* or Dukas's *The Sorcerer's Apprentice*. All of these experiences contributed to my sense of movement, but as yet I lacked an inner core or unifying force.

The center I needed began to develop in a very unexpected way. In order to get to my dance class in downtown Haifa, I had to ride a city bus which lumbered down the winding roads of Mt. Carmel. The bus had leather straps for passengers to hold on to while it went over rough spots, but I refrained from using them, preferring instead to stand freely in the aisle to try to keep my balance. Why? I wanted to meet the challenge of having to constantly adjust my posture and alignment to adapt to the moving bus. While the bus was turning, accelerating, or braking to a halt, I would bend my knees, widen my stance, or breathe down into my pelvic floor.

My dance studies were interrupted by two years of compulsory military service. I served in the army, developing sites for future kibbutzim. (A Hebrew word meaning "living in a type of commune.") When I was discharged, I was in my early twenties and eager to continue my dance training.

First, I needed to find a good teacher. I found an excellent one. Her name was Katia Michaeli, and she had come from Europe where she had once been a member of the company of a great pioneer of modern dance, Mary Wigman. Through training with Ms. Michaeli (who was also an Alexander technique teacher), I developed a rich sense of space, diagonals, and movement as well as basic theories, principles, and techniques of modern dance.

Somehow, throughout all this, I still felt that I was merely imitating others and not being true to myself. I needed to be authentic. I wanted what I was doing to arise out of universal truth, not reflecting the personality and philosophy of every teacher under whom I had studied. What I needed was a teacher who could help me find myself and my own unique expression. Ultimately, this led me to become the teacher I could not find.

Once again, still living in Israel, I came into contact with the Feldenkrais method. As Feldenkrais had a center in Israel, his method of re-education of the nervous system through movement awareness was readily available to me. For five years, I was absorbed in this method, among others, as I worked toward discovering my own movement.

In time, I became a certified teacher of human movement and dance. This later enabled me to incorporate my own knowledge of movement into other techniques of dance expression.

In the early 1980s, I came to the United States. I studied massage and other body techniques in order to physically contact the body systems and have personal, direct dialogue with them. I was introduced to Thera-Band® in 1982 in massage school. I tried it, but I was not too impressed with its narrow tube and the lack of support for the body part I was exercising. Then, in 1990, I attended a week-long workshop for dance teachers, where I used Thera-Band® again. This time the band was wider and much easier to use. Once I held it, ideas flowed. I began to develop exercises using the band while working with dancers at the Pinellas County Center for the Arts in St. Petersburg, Florida.

After eight years of teaching in Florida, I again felt a need to seek and search for greater depth. In 1991, I came across a wonderful guide named Bonnie Bainbridge Cohen—a teacher so intuitive and so profound that she evoked in me the process of inquiring and of learning to make distinctions among people's thinking, actions, and movements.

I hope to transfer some of the experience I have gained to you, the reader, as I share with you a safe and healthy technique of strengthening and stretching muscles with the aid of an elastic device called the Thera-Band®.

Noa Spector-Flock, 2001

Introduction

Introduction

The focus of this book is an exercise program which will teach you how to contract a specific muscle while lengthening it. This eccentric contraction (explained later) will integrate the movement of a certain muscle with the surrounding joints and muscles in that area, in order to involve the whole body and to create harmonious movement.

The contraction occurs while lengthening and stretching the fibers, yet the number of participating fibers decreases. Having less fiber share the load increases tension. Consequently, the overload stress and tension create greater stretch on the working fibers, resulting in enhanced flexibility.

The program will improve your sensory motor skills, enhancing coordination, strength and flexibility. Kinesthetic awareness will increase. The exercises will help you learn how to initiate movement from the larger and stronger muscles within the center of the body—which creates efficient movement—and let it continue through to the smaller muscles in the extremities. This order will result in more efficient and more delicate movement for expression.

Why would dancers be interested in the *Get Stronger by Stretching* program? Besides the more general benefits, dancers will develop the use of the psoas in lifting the leg (hip flexion). They will be able to extend their legs higher, and hold them longer. Low back stability will increase, thereby decreasing the possibility of pain and injury. By increasing the use of the lattisimus dorsi in correct body placement and arm usage, the back will stay wider, and arm movement will have better strength, control and coordination.

This exercise program will introduce you to Thera-Band®, an elastic device that can prepare you for any athletic activity. (See the "All About Thera-Band®" section on page 2.) Using the band during your warm-up simultaneously provides you with increased strength, flexibility, and circulation. As a result, *Get Stronger by Stretching with Thera-Band®* can be beneficial for all athletes, including dancers, swimmers, gymnasts, skiers, runners, etc., as well as for non-athletes who are looking for toned and fit bodies.

How This Book Is Organized

This book is divided into two chapters. Chapter 1 explains whole body movement. It contains discussions on stretching and strengthening, body alignment, and breathing. Chapter 2 is divided into muscle groups and areas, which will gain additional length and strength through proper attention and exercise using the body as a whole system. The exercises start at an easy level and build to a more difficult level by changing the position of the body or by increasing the complexity of the exercise. A brief conclusion expresses my hope for what you, the reader, will have gained from doing the exercises in this book.

All About Thera-Band®

What is Thera-Band®?

Thera-Band® is an elastic band used in exercising for improving strength, range of motion, and cooperation of muscle groups. It is part of a more general group of exercise devices called "resistance bands" or "resistive exercise bands." These bands both support and challenge your body as they stretch and return to unstretched length during exercise.

A latex Thera-Band® is six inches wide. A latex-free band is four inches wide and its resistive strength is similar to the latex Thera-Band®.

In this book, all exercises are demonstrated with a six-foot length of Thera-Band®.

The strength of Thera-Band® is indicated by a color code: tan (thinnest), yellow, red, green, blue, black, silver, and gold (the thickest and the newest addition). For example, based on the chart below, if you stretch one foot of the silver band to two feet (100% elongation), you will produce thirteen pounds of force. As your strength increases, you should move up to the next band. If you find that the silver band is too strong for you, you may opt to work with one of the thinner bands first. Because of this coding system, Thera-Band® gives at-a-glance proof of progress from one level to another.

% Elongation	50%	100%	150%	200%	250%
Yellow	2	3	4	5	6
Red	2.5	4	5	6	7
Green	3	5	6.5	8	9.5
Blue	4.5	7	9	11	13.5
Black	6.5	9.5	12.5	15	17.5
Silver	8.5	13	17	21	25.5
Gold	14	21.5	27.5	33.5	40

Getting acquainted with Thera-Band®

First, examine the band. Hold it in your hands. Does it lay comfortably in your hand? What color is it? How thick is it? How wide? Sense its texture, softness, and smoothness. Note the "chocolate smell" that rises from it. Take time to play with it. Notice its resistance: The resistance increases as the band is stretched and decreases as the band releases.

Experiment with the idea of isolating each of your arms from your torso. Next, combine the two and try to involve the torso with the movements of the arm. Now you are using more of yourself—the muscles of your torso and the muscles of your arms. You are thereby creating more flow. You are moving with integrated movement that will appear graceful.

Use of the band

The exercises in this book do not require any additional apparatus. However, if you prefer, the Hygenic Corporation (which produces the Thera-Band®) also produces the Thera-Band® Door Anchor, used to secure one end of the band for exercise. It isn't advisable to tie the exerciser to a door-knob or to "close" it in a door; this leads to early breaking. The Thera-Band® Exercise Handles and Assist can be used to grasp the exercisers. These can be used as an alternative to the band "loops" for some of the arm exercises, if desired. To connect to the legs or arms, use the Thera-Band® Extremity Strap.

Care of the band

The band can be damaged by extreme heat or sunlight. It should be stored in its package or in a dark place, such as a drawer, after each use. To keep the band soft and supple, sprinkle it with talcum powder or corn starch.

Why Thera-Band®?

At present, Thera-Band® is the only resistive exercise band endorsed by the American Physical Therapy Association. The Association's endorsement covers Thera-Band® latex and latex-free exercise bands and Thera-Band® exercise tubing.

APTA's endorsement can be likened to the Good Housekeeping Seal of Approval. It tells physical therapy professionals and the world at large that the Association has reviewed a particular product and feels that it is a good product. Thera-Band® products are used by physical therapists and other healthcare professionals as tools for conditioning, rehabilitation, and strength-building, and they have an excellent reputation for quality and effectiveness.

Thera-Band® is a well-established product, having been used during physical therapy and rehabilitation for years before the sports industry recognized its power for both strengthening and stretching. Because it is used in physical therapy and rehabilitation, it is available either through local medical supply stores or on the Internet.

Many resistance bands on the market are either too short or too narrow to be used in *Get Stronger by Stretching* exercises. Others are sold only in fixed form—that is, as a loop, figure-eight, or with wider sections for gripping.

Thera-Band® offers eight color-coded strengths, providing you with a more refined, graded system with easy-to-adapt-to progression from one level to the next. These Thera-Band® resistance values and the color progression are specific to the brand, and cannot be applied to other brands. There is no published research demonstrating the specific resistance levels or performance characteristics of other brands.

No other elastic resistive exerciser has been studied more extensively than Thera-Band® bands. Thera-Band® resistive exercisers have been clinically proven in use for more than 15 years to improve strength, range of motion, balance, and functional activities in many different patient populations. The Thera-Band® Academy also provides research and education for the use of all Thera-Band® products. The Thera-Band® exercisers are backed by the Hygenic Corporation, manufacturer of Thera-Band® products.

Why use a band instead of stretch tubing?

Although resistance tubing has the same stretch and strengthening potential as stretch bands, it does not work well with many exercises in this book.

Stretch bands lie flat against your body during exercises and stay in place, while tubing tends to roll with your moves. Tubing is also uncomfortable during exercises in which you lie down or stand on the band.

Where can I buy Thera-Band®?

Thera-Band® is available either through local medical supply stores, the Internet, or author Noa Spector-Flock.

THROUGH THERA-BAND® DEALERS:

Thera-Band® is manufactured by The Hygenic Corporation. You can contact the company directly to find a dealer near you. The following information is accurate as of 2001. Updated information is always on the company's website, <www.thera-band.com>.

In the United States or Canada:
1-800-321-2135
Monday–Friday: 8 a.m.–5 p.m. ET
The Hygenic Corporation
1245 Home Avenue
Akron, Ohio 44310

Outside the United States:
330-633-8460
330-633-9359 (fax)
Thera-Band GmbH Mainzer
Landstrasse 19
D-65589 Hadamar, Germany
+49 6433 91640;
+49 6433 9164 (fax)

THROUGH THE INTERNET:

Fitness Wholesale is a large distributor for Thera-Band®. Their web address for Thera-Band® is <www.fwonline.com/tbands.htm>

An Internet search using the keyword "Thera-Band" will list several other websites offering sales of Thera-Bands®.

FROM THE AUTHOR:

You may also purchase Thera-Band® directly from Noa Spector-Flock, through her e-mail address, <noanik8@att.net> or by telephone at 1-727-345-2570.

5

How much does Thera-Band® cost?

The cost of buying a six-foot length of Thera-Band®, the size used in the exercises in *Get Stronger by Stretching*, varies depending on where you buy it and what strength it is. Some websites are 50% higher than the prices available on the Fitness Wholesale website. Thera-Band® goes up in price as it gains strength, so you will pay more for a black roll than a yellow roll to cover the cost of the increase in material thickness.

Thera-Band® is available in three-band packages at two strengths. The Light Band Kit contains one each of yellow, red, and green bands. The Heavy Band Kit contains one each of blue, black, and silver.

Latex-free bands are available at Fitness Wholesale either in 25-yard rolls or by the foot. Their prices are similar to the latex Thera-Band®.

Frequently asked questions about Thera-Band® from the Thera-Band® Academy

Thera-Band® Academy is an organization that does research and development regarding Thera-Band®. Members are located throughout the world.

The following questions and answers are based on Thera-Band® Academy's "Frequently Asked Questions" on its website.

ELASTIC

Q. *What are the bands and tubing made of?*

A. Thera-Band® resistive bands are made of natural rubber latex made into sheets and tubing. Latex-free Thera-Band® resistive bands are made of synthetic rubber. The trademarked colors indicate the resistance levels.

Q. *What forces are produced by the bands?*

A. The force produced by bands is directly related to elongation. Each color will provide a specific amount of resistance at the same percent elongation, regardless of initial resting length. For example a 1-foot piece stretched to 2 feet (100% elongation) will have the same force as a 2-foot piece of the same color stretched to 4 feet. The force slowly increases as the band or tube is stretched.

A chart comparing the different colors is included in the "What is Thera-Band®" at the beginning of this section.

Q. *How do bands compare to free weights (such as dumbbells)?*
A. Elastic resistance has different properties from free weights, in that elastic resistance doesn't rely on gravity to produce force. Therefore, multiple patterns, speeds, and motions can be exercised with elastic resistance. Since the resistance increases with elongation, bands cannot be labeled with an absolute resistance level (e.g., yellow = 1 pound).

Bands also provide graduated resistance so that you have more control of how much resistance you are using. In addition, your body does not have to shift from zero resistance to a specific weight all at once. It experiences a gradual shift as the band is stretched during the exercise.

Q. *Do elastic bands provide similar results compared to free weights?*
A. Yes. Elastic resistance has been proven to be as effective as free weights in developing strength. Elastic bands are often substituted for free-weight exercises.

Q. *Doesn't the force increase at the end range, not allowing me to complete a full range of motion?*
A. As with any resistive exercise, elastic resistance must be used properly. While the force of the bands does increase with elongation, the "strength curve" of elastic resistance is physiologically similar to human joint strength curves. This provides less torque at the beginning and end ranges, where the muscles can't produce as much torque.

Q. *How many repetitions will the bands withstand?*
A. Elastic bands can last for a very long time with proper care and use. Thera-Band® elastic bands have been tested at more than 10,000 repetitions without any breakage.

Q. *How long can I stretch the bands?*
A. We don't recommend stretching beyond 300% elongation. The bands are more susceptible to breaking with greater than 500% elongation (for example, stretching a 1-foot piece to 6 feet), and the resistance increases sharply after 500%.

Q. *Why do the bands break, and what precautions should I take?*
A. With normal daily use, the exercisers should last for many months. However, they won't last forever. They may break if stretched beyond 500% or if they are used with small tears or abrasions. These small tears and abrasions usually occur at the "connection point" of the band to an attachment device. Therefore, always inspect the band (particularly near the connection) before use. *Get Stronger by Stretching* does not require any attachment devices. However, should you need or prefer them, it is recommended that you use the

Thera-Band® Door Anchor, Exercise Handle, and Assist for connection. Be aware that jewelry, fingernails, and other sharp objects may cause small tears or abrasions.

Always protect the eyes during exercise with elastic bands. Be sure to keep the band away from the eyes when stretching so that it does not snap back and hit you in the face. The bands are used for neck strengthening, so just be careful when using it around the face. Eyewear is not required.

Q. *When should I replace my bands?*

A. Always inspect your band for signs of wear, including small tears, abrasions, or cracks before use. Pay particular attention to the connection point. Always replace a band with any sign of wear. With heavy use, such as in a physical therapy clinic, bands should be replaced every one-to-two months. The bands will not last forever, and will experience normal wear and tear with extended use. However, they should be safe to use as long as there are no visible signs of wear.

The exact time for replacement varies depending on the number of sets, repetitions, and exercises performed, as well as how much it is stretched and how long it is in storage. With average use, the Thera-Band® Academy estimates that an exercise band would last more than 30 sessions—about 4 months. This would be much longer if the band is taken care of.

Q. *Can they be used in a chlorine pool?*

A. Yes, but the band will deteriorate at a quicker rate due to the chlorine. After each use in the pool, rinse the bands in tap water and hang them to dry.

Q. *What is the shelf life of Thera-Band® bands?*

A. When kept in a cool, dark environment, the bands should last for many years. However, use, exposure to temperature extremes, chlorine, and sunlight decrease the shelf life.

Q. *Why and under what circumstances is it better to prescribe latex-free Thera-Band® bands over standard latex Thera-Band® bands?*

A. The regular Thera-Band® resistive bands contain natural rubber latex. Latex allergies occur in a small percentage of the population (about 5–10%). When patients indicate latex allergy or sensitivity, they should use the latex-free bands. Also, patients with spina bifida tend to be more at-risk for latex allergy. Anyone using the latex bands who experiences an allergic reaction (such as redness or swelling on the skin near the band) should use the latex-free bands.

Q. *Can Thera-Band® bands be purchased powder free?*

A. The powder is used to keep the product from sticking to itself during manufacturing. The powder will be removed with normal use, and is not necessary for proper functioning of the product. Thera-Band® latex-free bands, however, do not contain powder.

Q. *Can I purchase single lengths of bands to replace the one I have?*

A. Yes. Replacements are available in light and heavy packs of three bands or tubes. Contact Customer Service for a dealer or retailer near you (1-800-321-2135). Author Noa Spector-Flock sells six-foot lengths of silver (1-727-345-2570 or <noanik8@att.net>).

Can I contact the Thera-Band® Academy?

If you have any questions for the Academy or want to find out what information it provides, it can be reached through its website at <http://www.thera-bandacademy.com>.

"Get Stronger by Stretching" and Pilates

How do the exercises in this book compare to the Pilates method developed by Joseph H. Pilates?

The full-body Thera-Band® system developed by Noa Spector-Flock in many ways parallels, and is complementary to the Pilates system. Both programs . . .

- Combine physical and mental conditioning to tone the muscles, gain strength and flexibility, and achieve the look desired.
- Utilize eccentric contraction, meaning the muscles contract and gain strength while they are being lengthened (rather then shortened). This contraction of the muscle on the lengthening phase creates a look that many people strive for—strong and lean.
- Pay special attention to the center of the body. The movements originate in the pelvic area and are carried to the extremities.
- Use mental concentration and controlled movement to enable the person to center the body, learn precision movement, and, with practice, achieve a harmonious flow of movement.
- Emphasize proper breathing and relaxation.

The elasticity and resistance supplied by the Thera-Band® is similar to that of the springs in Pilates equipment. But the Thera-Band® exercises in this book, like Pilates mat work (and unlike Pilates machine work), require only a mat.

Before You Start

What will you find in this book?

You will find exercises that deal with different muscle groups in the body. These exercises don't just strengthen or stretch muscles alone, but combine both elements. The process you will learn (mentioned in the Introduction) is called "eccentric contraction," which lengthens the muscle as you work it, thus making it stronger.

My main purpose in this book is to give you, the reader, an understanding of how to develop an "intelligent" body through proper breathing, posture, and the right exercise attitude. I hope to achieve this by emphasizing where to initiate the movement, and how to develop the exercise into an efficient movement that uses the correct muscles with the right amount of tension in them.

You can gain the most from this book if you follow these basic approaches:

1. START CAUTIOUSLY.

Use the exercises in this book with caution. Consult your doctor if you have any questions. Have a complete physical checkup before starting this or any new fitness program, especially if you have medical conditions such as high blood pressure, varicose veins, bursitis, or arthritis.

2. WORK SLOWLY.

This means *very slowly*, for two reasons:

A. The slower you work, the more control you will have over the movement.

B. By slowing down, you can pay closer attention and learn *how* to do the exercises. You will learn which patterns you are already moving in by habit. Once you know this, you will be able to change old patterns and learn new ones.

3. USE YOUR BREATHING.

Keep the breathing rhythmic and constant. As a general rule, movements are most efficient if they are executed while you are breathing evenly and continuously.

Many times we find ourselves holding our breath on the effort part of a movement. However, any movement will be easier to do if you conscientiously exhale as the effort is being carried out. For example, sitting on the floor with your legs straight in front of you, fully exhale as you lower your torso behind you toward the floor by using your abdominal muscles. If you exhale while humming a song, you can be sure that you are not holding your breath. While down, pause to inhale; then again, fully exhale as you resume a sitting position. In other words, you should exhale on both the extension (exertion) and flexion (return) of the movement.

4. PAY ATTENTION.

Become aware of what you are doing so it does not become mechanical. Establish the intention of making the connection between body and mind. The holistic approach (body, mind, and spirit) will bring better and faster results to your physical appearance and well-being. Always be aware of how the process is taking place and the parts of the body that are involved. For example, by retracting the abdominal muscles you are able to raise your leg higher because of the psoas muscle contraction.

5. MAINTAIN BODY ALIGNMENT.

A. When bending your knees, whether you are sitting, standing, or lying down, you must create a straight, imaginary line that runs from the hip to the center of the knees, then to a point on the side border of the second toe between the second and third toe. This will ensure that you develop all sides of your leg and foot equally, not using one muscle over the others, which will prevent stress. It also avoids eversion/inversion (twisting of the foot) that creates overload and strain. (See photo on the next page.)

B. While in a sitting position, place yourself on top of your "sitting bones" (your ischial tuberosities), neither in front nor behind them. Stack your vertebrae above them to create a balance so that the bones support you, rather than just using your back muscles.

C. When inhaling, or when lifting your arms over your head, keep the rib cage aligned (tucked in) and not sticking out in front. Imagine the ribs to be like a closed umbrella rather than an open one. This avoids unnecessary stress on the vertebrae in your mid-back.

D. Keep your head as a continuation of the back. Do not let the chin protrude forward; rather, bring it downward slightly and toward the spine.

E. Keep 180° between the shoulders so that your collarbone is parallel to the floor. The shoulders should not be elevated but should be open. Your muscles in your upper chest (pectoralis) need to be long and relaxed so that the shoulders don't roll forward. Work on your balance between forward and backward (anterior and posterior).

F. Never lock your knees or elbows. When you lengthen your legs, think of lengthening them from the back of the leg while pulling your heels out away from you.

6. USE CAUTION.

Use your comfort as a guide when exercising the knees, lower back, and shoulder joints.

A. *Knees*

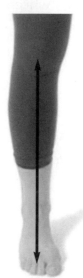

If you have an injury to your knee, you may avoid undue pressure by tying the band above the knee instead of below it. When doing leg exercises with such movements as bringing a body part away from the center line of the body (abduction), bringing a body part closer to the center line of the body (adduction), and turn in/ turn out, always bend your knees very slightly to prevent hyperextension. This is especially important if you have experienced this problem in the past.

B. *Lower Back*

For exercises done while lying on the spine (supine) on the floor, you should NEVER release the lower back in an arch greater than your normal posture. Holding and supporting the abdominal muscles against the lower back will keep the lower back from arching. Exhaling on the effort in all exercises will also help. The transversus abdominis muscles will be engaged and contracted against the back, and all around. This creates a hollow sensation and look to the abdominal area and is different from a pelvic tilt.

When in a standing position, allow the lower back to drop down with a very small pelvic tilt (hardly noticeable, mostly felt) to the front, so the spine is kept as straight as possible. Your knee position will also affect the lumbar area, so again, bend your knees slightly.

C. *Shoulder Joints*

People with restrictions in their shoulder joints will have to use less resistance and increase the slack in the band. To improve, do only a very small portion of each movement. Try to isolate the feeling of lengthening the arm outward to "create space" in the socket before you actually lift the arm. You should also learn to use the muscles of the back to support the arms so that most of the effort will fall upon the bigger muscles (trapezius, latissimus dorsi, and the rhomboids), which are better suited for that function. (See 2.1.5 on page 41 and 2.1.9 on page 42.)

7. MAINTAIN BODY POSITION.

Pay attention to the position described for each of the exercises that follow for best results. For example, while exercising the abdominal area, it is important to maintain the arms in the specified position to work the muscle that connects the arm to the back (latissimus dorsi).

8. WORK SIMPLY.

Do not try to look nice by adding unnecessary gestures to the movement. Pay attention to how you use your body for the movement. Know the origin of the movement and how it is developed through the body to other parts. This will create a fully developed sequence that will be both efficient and in harmony with proper body movement.

9. CREATE SPACE.

Throughout the book, the expression "making space in the joint" is used. This means, when you start to move a limb, do not push it into the joint in order to move it. Instead, try to do the opposite: create the sensation of lengthening the limb out of the joint before even contracting the muscle to move. One good way to achieve this is to exhale while creating the lengthening sensation. This is a safe way to exercise and will not irritate arthritic conditions. For example, when lifting your arm above your head, think of the arm being pulled out from the shoulder joint before you lift it.

10. WORK DEEPLY.

Do not move only your extremities to "get some exercise." Rather, you should pay attention to your inner sensations. Move using the big muscles in the center of your body to initiate the movement; then make space in the joints to move the extremities.

11. WORK EVENLY.

Remember we move in habitual patterns. Our bodies are not symmetrical and, therefore, are not symmetrically strong, long, or flexible. Pay attention to this, and work as evenly as possible to create new patterns. In this way, the load of the work can be shared more equally on the muscles, ligaments, tendons, and joints in the body.

12. BE AWARE OF YOUR RESISTANCE LEVEL.

The shorter the distance is between your hands on the band, the more resistance you will have. Doubling the band doubles the resistance. You may also decide to move ahead to a stronger band when necessary, in order to increase your level of resistance. (Be sure to check the Thera-Band® section starting on page 2 for more information about the exercise bands used in these exercises.)

13. FOLLOW THESE SIMPLE RULES:

- Keep the band away from young children and pets.
- Cover sensitive areas of your skin or hairy areas of your body to prevent pinching or pulling.
- Secure long hair on top of the head.
- Keep the wrists straight to create a continuous line from forearm to hand.
- Always pull the band away from the body; be careful not to hit your face.
- Always be in control while pulling or releasing to the starting position.
- Always check the band for possible damage before use.

Starting a Workout

If you are a beginner or a person who would like to get back into shape again, I suggest that you follow the whole body program for a while (see Appendix D on page 171). The general rule is to start with a few repetitions and build up. That means that when I teach, depending on the group ability we may start with 2 repetitions and build to 4, 5, and 6. A more experienced person could start with 4 repetitions. With the longer exercises, 2 or 3 repetitions will be enough because that body part that is being used gets really tired after awhile.

When you feel that your body "knows" the exercises—that is, when you feel strong enough for 12–15 repetitions and are fluent in your movement—then you may try another combination. Once you work with the book and fully understand its intent, you may build your own program according to your creativity and needs.

If you are a professional dancer or athlete who exercises with the band, you may choose to concentrate on a specific area of the body one day (the upper body, for example), employing the appropriate exercises for it, and then concentrate on a different area the next day (like the lower body). This will rest the muscle groups and you will not overwork any one area of the body.

The main point is this: Each person should assess what is appropriate for his or her body and not feel that this program is etched in stone.

You may use the exercises in this book as a means of warming-up for other activities, taking into account that you "create space" in your joints. Use your breath at all times, and move in the directions the body is designed to move in. Do not push against joints, tendons, or ligaments.

1. Read through each exercise, noting the photographs. The exercises are generally explained only to one side so you can learn how to do them; it is expected that you will also repeat them to the other side. The abbreviations "R" and "L" are used in place of "right" and "left," respectively.

2. Once you understand the exercise, do it once on the specified side to get the basic feel for it, then repeat it to the opposite side so your body will be worked equally on both sides.

3. As you get stronger, gradually increase the number of repetitions you do until you reach 12–15 times on each side. This way, you can build up muscle endurance—the ability of the muscles to sustain work over time and through the repetition of effort. Using 60–80% of your total muscle power will be sufficient to increase your strength.

The band will offer the resistance you need to gain both strength and endurance. In fact, an endurance baseline may be established by doing just 6–8 repetitions of each exercise regularly. You can gauge the amount of resistance you are using and the rate of your improvement by the distance of the band stretch. The shorter the band, the greater the resistance will be (you may mark the band with a pen). Refer to the color code chart on page 2. (Thera-Band® Academy cautions against "shortening up" the band too much because it changes the usefulness of the band. Instead, they suggest increased repetitions or moving up to the next color band.)

When you design your program, make sure you keep in mind the needs of your particular sport or specialty. (For example, runners would have no need to concentrate on the outward rotation of the hip, to the degree ballet dancers would.) Three sample workouts, located at the end of the book, are provided for you to use as a model for how to design your own individual workout routine. The sample workouts are a general three-part whole-body program, and two specific programs for dance conditioning and swim conditioning.

How to tie your Thera-Band®

Before you start to work with your Thera-Band®, hold the band in your hand. Feel how smooth it is and how compact it becomes when folded for storage. Experience the chocolate smell from the talcum that helps keep your band healthy—and which you should use as well from time to time.

To make a loop, sit down and put one end of the band under the sole of your foot. Make a very simple tie. Leave a little space between the loop and your foot so you don't pinch yourself, and leave about eight inches on the end of the band. Make another tie—a simple flat tie.

All that is left is to push the knot down to secure it. You should have about four inches left on the end of the band. The pushing down and extra space at the end insure that the band won't roll or become unknotted.

You need to have loops on both ends of the band for some exercises in this book, so be sure to tie the other end as well.

Conclusion

I have constructed the exercises so that they reach and work the muscles from different angles. For example, consider an exercise that flexes and extends the thigh and knee. The advanced version would be to rotate the leg out while repeating the same exercise, which would affect additional (or entirely different) fibers of the muscle.

My main goal is to create strength and length in your body equally, so that both qualities support and balance each other. More than that, my vision is that your body will then integrate efficiency and harmony of movement. This is why I chose exercises involving muscle groups and integrating areas. I hope that by following the instructions described, you will learn how to initiate movement from a strong muscle in the center of your body (for example, the psoas, which connects the upper lumber spine with the head of the femur and bridges the lower back with the lower extremities), and to include more muscles as the movement develops and expands.

It is important to be aware of what and how the exercise is carried out—of the process taking place and the body parts that are involved. For example, it is helpful to realize that by retracting the abdominal muscles (i.e., originating and initiating the contraction with the psoas muscle) it becomes easier to raise the leg high. The holistic approach—body, mind, and spirit—brings better and faster results not only to your physical appearance, but also, to your well-being.

This way you can experience the full sensation of integrated whole body movement.

Enjoy!

Noa Spector-Flock

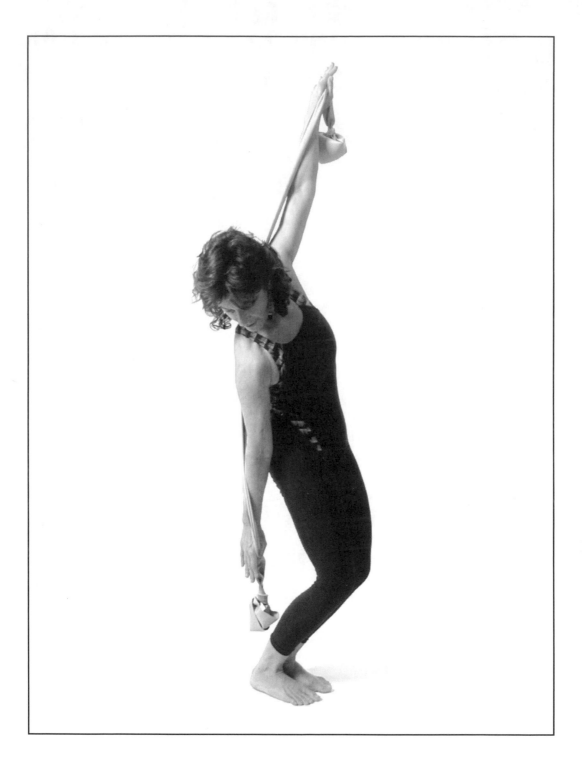

Chapter 1
Chapter One

ACHIEVING WHOLE BODY MOVEMENT

Organic learning is essential. It can also be therapeutic in essence. It is heal-
thier to learn than to be a patient or even be cured. Life is a process, not a
thing. And processes go well if there are many ways to influence them. We
need more ways to do what we want than the one we know—even if it is a
good one in itself.

> — Moshe Feldenkrais
> *The Elusive Obvious* (1981: 29)

Stretching and Strengthening

Dancers are constantly stretching their muscles to increase their flexibility and their range of motion, especially in the hip socket, spine, and feet. However, strength is the other side of flexibility. Too much flexibility in the muscles without adequate strength results in uncontrolled mobility, loose joints, and overall weakness. Too often, this condition results in injury. On the other hand, too much strength without much flexibility limits the range of motion. For a muscle to become stronger, you need to increase the frequency and the intensity of an exercise, and lengthen the the period of time in which it is complete. This can be achieved by using the Thera-Band®. For the muscle to become more flexible, it must be stretched for a specific length of time.

The ideal situation creates a balance between stretching and strengthening that provides many benefits:

1. The range of motion (ROM) increases and continues to evolve as the strength and stretch in the body also increase. In other words, we will assume that you start with the ability to stretch your leg to the side to a certain point. It is only after you acquire the strength to hold it there, that you can work on stretching your leg higher. Flexibility is great only if you have the strength to use what you have while you are moving.

2. A combination of exercises that both stretch and strengthen the muscles will promote a better blood supply—and therefore, a better oxygen supply—to the muscles and the organs. This means you will have a better workout on the day you exercise, and less soreness on "the morning after."

3. As we stretch the muscles, we will also elongate the fascia, which supports and holds the muscle fibers together, and connects the muscle groups.

4. By strengthening a muscle while contracting it eccentrically, we keep it long and flexible. This prevents injuries around the joint, such as ligament sprains, tendon strains, and partial joint dislocation (subluxation).

5. Muscle soreness usually occurs only in the early stages of an exercise program. As a person gets stronger and more flexible using the band, soreness is no longer a factor.

Definition of Terms

Types of Muscle Movement*

Muscles can be contracted, relaxed, or elongated. This happens on a chemical level as well as on a physical level. The changes in the muscle length are due to the thick and thin myofilament (actin and myosin) sliding along each other.

A CONTRACTION builds tension in the muscle fibers, generates movement, helps maintain posture, and produces body heat. Chemically, a contraction occurs when calcium is released into the muscle body.

RELAXATION is totally passive. When the muscle fibers receive no more impulses, they let go; they relax. In other words, there is no more generation of muscle tension because the calcium that was there has withdrawn.

ELONGATION can occur when a force outside a particular muscle is used. This force can be any of the following:

1. gravity

2. body motion

3. an antagonist muscle working in opposition to the muscle being activated (for example, the hamstring versus quadriceps)

4. another person or machine pulling on the body part.

With the Thera-Band®, we mostly contract eccentrically, meaning we will build tension while elongating the muscle. (See a more complete definition in next section.) The stretching combined with the resistance of the band makes the muscle stronger.

Types of Contractions

ISOMETRIC CONTRACTION

Isometric contraction occurs when the distance between each end of the muscle—the origin and the insertion—remains the same even though the muscle is contracting. Observers cannot see outer movement but the person engaging in that contraction will sense the muscle fibers are condensing or

---

*See Spector-Flock (2001) for more details.

extending, giving a different quality of sensation. This occurs when a muscle attempts to push or pull an object that is immovable.

ISOTONIC CONTRACTION

During isotonic contraction, outer (visible) movement does take place. Here the contracting muscle generates the tension, which is greater than the load on the muscle. Isotonic contraction includes two types, concentric contraction and eccentric contraction.

CONCENTRIC CONTRACTION

Concentric contraction occurs when the distance between each end of the muscle—the origin and the insertion—becomes smaller. In this shortening contraction, as the muscle shortens, the tension decreases. This compels more of the muscle fibers to participate in the pull. The whole muscle protects the connective tissue from soreness as it shares

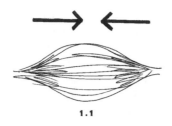

1.1

the workload. Lifting a heavy suitcase is an example of concentric contraction. Concentric contraction is used in opposition to eccentric contraction. For example, if the muscles on one side of a joint are concentricallly contracting, the muscles on the other side of the joint will be eccentrically contracting. (1.1)

ECCENTRIC CONTRACTION

For eccentric contraction to occur, the entire muscle group must work its full range of motion (ROM), and there must be a gradual emphasis on the negative phase of the work—the lowering phase of the resistance. Eccentric contraction is a lengthening contraction. It occurs when the contracting muscle fibers become more extended and the distance between each end of the muscle—the origin and the insertion—is increased. In eccentric contraction, few muscle fibers are capable of contracting individually. This puts much tension on the connective tissue, which may later relate to muscle soreness. In my clinical and classroom experience, I have found that soreness occurred only in the early stages of the program and as the person gets stronger and more flexible using the band, the soreness is no longer a factor. (1.2)

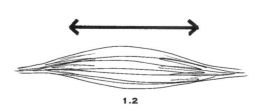

1.2

Types of Stretching

One way to understand stretching is from the range-of-motion (ROM) viewpoint. In this approach there are four ways to create exercise results:

PASSIVE

An outside force pushes or pulls a body part, such as a leg, while your entire body remains relaxed.

PASSIVE/ACTIVE

Passive/active stretch is similar to passive, except at the peak of the stretch, the position is held for a few seconds by a second person.

ACTIVE/ASSISTED

You stretch to your limits and then an outside force continues to stretch you further. Care, knowledge, and sensitivity must be exercised to avoid tearing a muscle or tendon.

ACTIVE

You use your own muscle power without outside aid. Active stretching can be either STATIC or BALLISTIC.

> STATIC is a slow steady stretch (as in yoga) during which the body is being stretched to the point where tightness is felt. You then hold the stretch for 2–30 seconds, depending on the approach. Holding the position allows the inner structure to respond gradually to the stretch/tension and the muscle relaxes. Using breath and exhaling into the stretch also enhance the stretch.

> BALLISTIC stretch occurs when the body part bounces or "pops" over the joint. The weight of the body or body part moving with speed builds up momentum with energy that causes tissue damage (micro damage), especially over time. Michael Alter explains that sudden or painful movement causes muscle contraction. As a result, ballistic stretching should be avoided.

The approach taken in this book is the active-static stretch. Some research may show that a combination of static and ballistic stretching could be the most beneficial, but ballistic stretching is known to cause injuries, especially to the tendons. It is very hard on the joints. My goal is to "create space" in the joints, which will avoid grinding and tension. Therefore, static stretching with the aid of the Thera-Band® will safely give you the results you are looking for—and much more.

Another method of stretching is P.N.F. Proprioreceptor Neuromuscular Facilitation, which is a type of stretching developed in the 1940s and designed to treat people with paralysis. The method uses the body's primitive muscle reflexes. Two of the techniques are:

1. CONTRACT-RELAX: You contract the muscle you want to stretch for 15 seconds. The golgi tendon registers the tension increase and causes autogenic inhibition, and that muscle will stretch further.

2. CONTRACT-RELAX-AGONIST-CONTRACT (CRAC): Contract-relax holding the contraction for 20 seconds. You pause for a second and then you contract the opposing muscle to be stretched. (For more details, see *reciprocal innervation* in Appendix A on page 165.)

Some Principles for Muscle Movement

We have a whole network of muscles, about 600 of them. Examples are cardiac (relating to the heart), visceral (in the walls of internal structures), and skeletal (attached to bones). Our muscles are either involuntary or voluntary. Voluntary muscles are the ones designed for controlled movement by using our nervous system.

Muscles are all arranged in sac-like wraps, covered by fascia, in different sizes and shapes, ready for the neurologic input intended to start movement. Skeletal muscles contract according to the "graded strength" principle. This means that they contract with varying degrees of strength at different times, which enables us to adjust from lifting a pen to lifting a full suitcase. This is different from the all-or-none rule on the fiber contraction level.

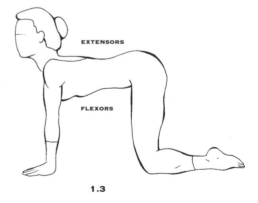

1.3

Skeletal muscles almost always work in groups. There is a coordinated action of several muscles for performing every movement. This means that when a prime muscle is contracting an opposing (antagonist) muscle relaxes.

At times there are muscles that work in a synergy to help the prime mover. This allows a dynamic tension, which means that if the front of the body has to flex (bend) forward to pick up a bag, the muscles in the back of the body have to let go, and even extend, to allow that motion. (1.3)

GRAVITY: Gravity calls us to "pay attention to the verticality of the body." This means that the skeleton needs to be aligned. In some of the exercises, such as leg work, I work against gravity using it in a dynamic way.

I tried to honor these principles by creating movements that combine muscle groups as we need them for daily function rather than trying to artificially isolate them. By doing so, the movements keep the natural joint motion, which in return helps to keep, or restore, joint health.

Body Alignment

Body alignment is the habitual way in which we each maintain our own body posture or placement. Personal body alignment can be acquired through

- imitation (e.g., baby watching parents),
- use or misuse of the body of which you are unaware (e.g., sitting for hours in a chair), and/or
- genetic defects (e.g., one leg longer than the other).

Good posture (alignment) is crucial to maintaining good health. It provides the appropriate starting point for any movement or posture desired. Proper alignment also eliminates unnecessary stress on muscles, tendons, bones, and joints. Standing becomes easier, breathing becomes freer, and movement becomes possible in any direction.

Good alignment eliminates unnecessary stress on the body and the body maintains uprightness in space against gravity. Bones are stacked one on top of another in a way that allows the weight to be directed through the bones that are specifically designed to carry the body's weight.

Good alignment allows the nervous system and the supporting deep muscles, fascias, tendons, and ligaments to give the support needed to free the muscles for movement. When the bones support the body weight, the muscles can relax and more easily contract when movement is desired. (See Ida P. Rolf's book *Rolfing: The Integration of Human Structures*, for more details.)

Good alignment also distributes balance between weight-bearing and weight-transferring areas of the skeleton. You need to find the right relationship between muscles that work as movers and antagonist muscles that oppose the movement, thus enabling you to move with ease and efficiency. For example, the muscles on all four sides of your lower leg work together in harmony, functioning in weight-transference, so that your ankle and foot can move as they were intended, as weight-bearers.

Personally, I believe that one of the ways we express ourselves in the world is in the posture and alignment we create through our lifetime. Our feelings, attitudes, and internal conversations about the outer world are factors that creates our posture. Heritage, repetitive movements, injuries, body structure, and such are the others.

My goal is to give you the opportunity to view posture as dynamic, to see that transition from posture to posture allows us to be alive in our body alignment. Alive—aware of who we choose to be mentally and spiritually that expresses itself in the physical body.

Planes of Movement

One of the ways to analyze muscle function and movement is to isolate the three distinct planes of the body (1.4):

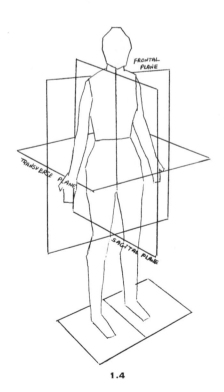

FRONTAL PLANE: division from one side of the body to the other, creating separate front and back regions; movement in this plane is sagittal (directly forward and backward).

SAGITTAL PLANE: division through the center of the body, creating two symmetrical halves; movement in this plane is frontal (with the face forward; e.g., lateral bend to the side).

HORIZONTAL PLANE: division of the body at the waistline into upper and lower regions; movement in this plane is rotation.

1.4

Looking at Your Own Body Alignment

When you check your body for good alignment, divide your body into right and left sides, comparing size and length of different body parts. You will also divide your body into front/back and lower/upper relationships.

The main body parts to check are:

- the feet position
- Achilles tendon alignment to the midline calf muscle
- behind the knees looking at the muscle bulk
- front of center kneecap aligned between second and third toe
- front and back of pelvis (1.6 and 1.7)
- skin creases along the side of the torso
- ribs
- spine deviation from center: right-to-left and forward/backward (1.5)
- shoulder level, and ear level (1.5)

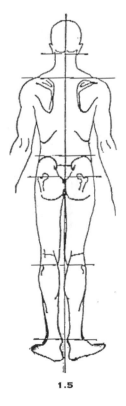

1.5

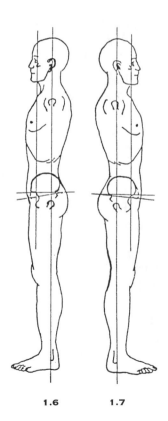

1.6   **1.7**

Compare one side with the other, looking for such conditions as one shoulder higher than the other, one knee turned inward, or one inner thigh muscle more or less developed than the other. As you practice observing, you will develop an "eye" for recognizing areas of muscles that are defined, as opposed to areas of weakness and low tonicity; areas with "moving energy" and areas with no "life."

The relationship between posture and skeletal structure is alive and ongoing throughout your lifetime. Most people find that their body structure mirrors and profoundly influences their posture. By opening up an awareness of body language—that is, by paying attention to how you do things: how you stand, sit, step, or adjust your balance—you will avoid body stiffening, inflexibility, imbalance, and/or pain in the soft tissues. You will become more dynamic.

EXAMPLES OF COMMON OF MISALIGNMENTS

1. The neck protrudes forward causing stress on the cervical vertebras. This causes the back (posterior) neck muscles to be contracted continuously and the front (anterior) neck muscles to be long and weak, causing imbalance that may lead to injury and pain. (1.8)

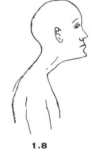

1.8

2. Knees turn in more than the feet. Stress is then placed on the tendons and ligaments on the side (lateral) aspects of the knee and the inner/ outer thigh muscles become under stress. The side muscles in the lower leg may build enough stress for you to sense pain. (1.9)

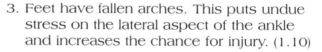

3. Feet have fallen arches. This puts undue stress on the lateral aspect of the ankle and increases the chance for injury. (1.10)

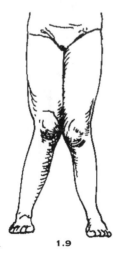

1.9

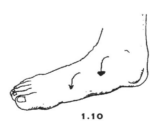

1.10

The human body is not a static structure; it is very dynamic and constantly moving. In order to adapt to each new position, good alignment continuously changes as the body keeps moving. Therefore, when thinking about posture, we should not relate it just to any one position, but to the relationships among body parts as they are moving. When we are able to move harmoniously from one point to another with the required effort—not more and not less—we are on the path toward better alignment.

The center of gravity in the body also changes as we move. Normally, our center of gravity is high, 1–2 inches (the width of four fingers) below the navel. This relatively high center of gravity enables us to move in a dynamic way. When the center of gravity in the body lowers (wide stance and bent knees), we become more stable and move more slowly.

There are specific tests for determining if you are in proper alignment. The Thomas test measures tightness of the pelvis (iliopsoas and rectus femoris muscles). The Ober test measures adductor tightness (ITB and gluteal muscles). The Tripod test measures the tightness of the hamstring muscle group and its effect on the pelvic tilt. There are many more tests.

The key point is this: If you try to maintain a position that seems to be good posture to you, and yet you are uncomfortable, your muscles are probably doing most of the work. You probably do not have enough skeletal support. Improvement will come when you start viewing your alignment as a dynamic process that allows your muscles and skeleton to work together in enhancing core stability involving the deep muscles in your torso.

For example, suppose you are sitting with your legs crossed in front of you. If you are unable to maintain the position for a long time, you may suffer from any of the following problems.

1. Your weight may not be on both sitting bones evenly, or it may be either in front of or behind the sitting bones. (1.11 and 1.12)

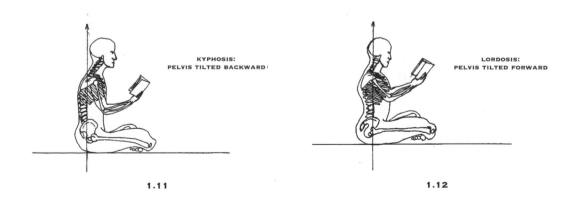

KYPHOSIS:
PELVIS TILTED BACKWARD

LORDOSIS:
PELVIS TILTED FORWARD

1.11   1.12

2. You may not be breathing down into your lower abdomen or lower back (where your floating ribs are), but may be breathing shallowly in your upper chest only.

3. Your weight may not be falling through the front of the second lumbar vertebra.

4. Your chest may be sinking back while your neck is pushed forward.

You will improve your body alignment by finding the place where the bones carry the body weight and the muscles are free to move. (1.13)

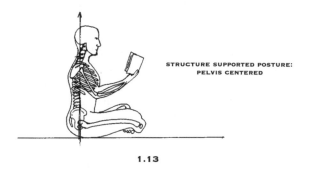

STRUCTURE SUPPORTED POSTURE:
PELVIS CENTERED

1.13

Breathing

Any time that we find ourselves under a physical demand, we may become somewhat aware of the way we are breathing. Our breathing patterns tend to change with our emotions. For example, we breath differently when we feel fear, hesitation, surprise, joy, happiness, or even when something simply interests us. Singers and dancers often have specific breathing techniques they must learn. We breath differently in different body positions—lying on one side (which puts pressure on one lung), sitting, standing, or even hanging upside-down.

Think of the rib cage as a container for the thoracic cavity, which holds the lungs. The heart sits in between them, to the left side of center. This explains why the left lung is slightly smaller than the right one, and why the bronchus of the left lung has only two main branches instead of three, as the right one has. (1.14)

The lungs help our body absorb oxygen into our cells when we inhale, and get rid of excess carbon dioxide when we exhale. They do not move on their own.

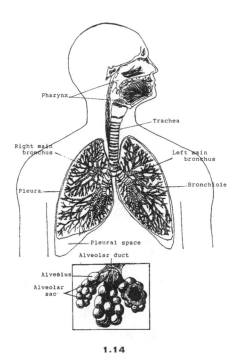

1.14

Breathing movement occurs in the muscles surrounding the lungs. The main muscle that initiates the breathing action and also performs 80% of the work is the diaphragm—a strong, thin muscle located between the thoracic and abdominal cavities. It is attached to the lower border of the rib cage (anterior, i.e., in the front) and all the way around to the spine (posterior, i.e., in the back). When we inhale, the diaphragm contracts by flattening downward into the abdomen, enlarging the thoracic cavity, and allowing atmospheric pressure to cause air to flow into the body from the outside.

Another muscle that contracts during inhalation is the intercostal muscle located between the ribs. Also, when we inhale deeply or forcefully exhale, other muscles, such as those around the shoulder, neck, and back, may also get involved.

Exhalation is a reverse process of inhalation: the muscles stop contracting and start relaxing. Air simply flows out of the trachea and the mouth or nose as the abdominal and thoracic muscles and organs return to their original positions.

Breathing is a key to well-being in many belief systems—not just physical well-being, but also mental and emotional. Each one of us can improve the way we breathe in order to benefit our health.

One of the things I stress most in this book is for you to keep your breath-

31

ing pattern steady and constant as you exercise, using the whole thoracic cavity—in front, in back, and along the sides, from the sternum down into the pelvis. Notice when your rhythm changes; it may be an indication of difficulty or an anticipation of effort. Check your body alignment and muscle relaxation between repetitions to be certain that there is no tension or exertion. If you find that you are starting to hold your breath, STOP! Go back to the beginning of the exercise, then start to exhale as you perform the movement. A simple test is to see if you can speak or sing as you exercise. If you can, then you are exhaling.

Adjust your workout to your abilities and needs, so that when you are finished, you feel invigorated rather than exhausted.

Head and Tailbone Relationship

The head and tailbone are at the two ends of the spine; therefore, it is very important that they work together. From the time that you were a baby, they each responded to the other naturally when you moved. For example, this is evident when you arched your neck and head, trying to crawl on your stomach (in the prone position) and later on your hands and knees. Chiropractors tend to utilize that principle in their work.

This relationship also can be seen when you work from the all-fours position (on your hands and knees). As you arch the spine, both the head and the tailbone will be directed up toward the ceiling. As the spine curves upward, both the head and tailbone will be directed down toward the floor. You can see this when a cat stretches as it wakes up.

For more information on the relationship of the head and tailbone, particularly during infancy and childhood, please refer to Bonnie Bainbridge Cohen's studies at the School for Body-Mind Centering, listed in the Bibliography at the end of this book. (1.15)

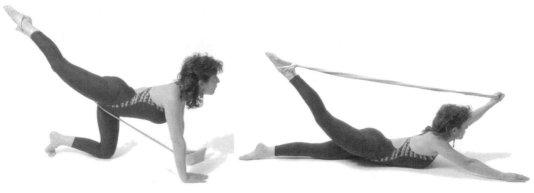

1.15

Awareness

Feldenkrais writes in his book *Awareness Through Movement*, "Awareness is consciousness together with a realization of what is happening within it or what is going on within ourselves while we are conscious" (Feldenkrais, 50). Having adequate awareness means that we know what it is we are doing while we are doing it.

Awareness is the strongest tool I know of that we have for relearning and reeducating ourselves. Awareness is the extra ingredient we should add to moving, thinking, sensing, and feeling. We learn to move as infants by imitation. We do movements mostly the way we learned them, and get into habits. As adults we can improve some habitual ways we move. This will enable us to understand and know how we do our movements, and how to do them with the least amount of strain and force.

Gaining awareness gives us the ability to choose. It also gives us access to the body/mind connection we all feel and know we have. For example, changing our body posture when we feel fear will result in altering our feeling to some extent. Change of mental focus can effect the intensity of pain, and positive thoughts can alter our mental state.

The avenues to body/mind connection are many. I hope that the journey through the physical realm I bring here will give you access to finding your connection. Although the intent here is to achieve a stronger and more flexible body, if you do the exercises with intention, attention, and awareness (mindfulness) you will get closer to your full potential, finding improvement in both body and mind.

Lessons from Life

#1 INTERCONNECTIONS

One hot summer afternoon, to escape from domestic drudgery, I went to a movie, little realizing the intellectual workout in store for me. Besides forcing me to think about major dilemmas of our time, the movie, *Mind Walk*, introduced me to a new term important in physics: interconnections. As a result of this term and the way it was used in the movie, I now look at people, things, and places with a somewhat new awareness. I now perceive how all of these relate to each other through vibrations of energy. I am discovering truth and comfort in knowing that I am related to all that I see, hear, feel, and touch—and in more subtle ways, such as the silver mercury that fills some of my teeth, or the material I am wearing.

Mind Walk featured three distinct types of people, each with a different outlook on life. There was the physicist, whose outlook was scientific yet holistic and avant-garde; the politician, who was pragmatic; and the poet/political speechwriter who represented the arts. A bridge was effected between the scientist and politician. It remained for the poet to remind us of the absolute necessity of emotions for a full, complete understanding of life function.

So there it is: function, force, and feeling, all integrated, all interconnected. Interconnections.

#2 SAFE/HEALTHY MOVEMENT

It is possible to actually believe that dancers or athletes are somehow more than normal when we see them in competition or performance. Their abilities amaze us. However, behind the outward appearances and without safe practices, pain and injury are often the price of excellence.

We sometimes forget the human structure—the shape of the joints, the length of the ligaments and tendons—and try to reach the aesthetic beauty that our culture and the tradition of classical ballet has set for us. We strive for the speed and agility of many sports. By knowing the body movement capability from within, along with realistic assessment of capabilities, we may be able to minimize damage to our bodies. We should "create space" in the joints before we move and use deep muscles in a three-dimensional fashion in all that we do.

#3 BEING ONE WITH NATURE

Once, while serving in the Israeli army, I was in an army settlement that was soon to be turned into a civil community. I took a late walk one night outside the security fence, not thinking of the danger or the consequences.

The next morning, there was a gathering of people in the central dining hall, and their emotions were very stirred. I soon learned that the Bedouin who walked the borders that morning had found footprints. Just by looking at them, he could tell that they were left by a five-foot, two-inch-tall female who was about 20 years old. I knew there was nothing left for me to do. So with a smile and a guilty conscience I stepped forward.

I then spent years looking to discover even part of what he never forgot from his years of living in the desert and being one with nature and its courses.

#4 CHAIRS

Do I need my hands to get up from a chair?

It depends from which end of life you look at it. For a young child, it is easy. For an elderly person, it may be a major effort. (Just look at all the TV advertisements for automatic chairs that lift you up from them!)

As I see the task, it all boils down to a shift of weight and correct timing. It is not a matter of being "strong" enough to pull yourself up, but of how to use your body correctly.

Start moving your upper body toward the edge of the chair with your sitting bones touching the edge and your feet flat on the floor about as far apart as your pelvic width. Start exploring by shifting your upper-body weight forward and backward, then side to side. Find your personal comfort zone. Find when discomfort starts to creep in. Notice that when you shift your weight forward, your heels dig into the floor to have full contact. What happens to your abdominal muscles then?

Now pay attention to what happens to your neck and chin as you shift your weight forward. Can you feel the curvature in your neck also going forward?

When you shift enough weight forward, your pelvis will elevate and rotate a bit forward, the curvature in your neck will increase, the weight will be over your feet (through the side border of the second toe between the second and third toe), and you will be lifting out of the chair to a "chimpanzee position." From there to an upright standing position, the distance is short.

#5 YOUR WALK "SPEAKS"

I remember days in college when it was just too much and I needed air. I would go to one of my favorite places to escape from stress: the beach. But even while I was there, my interest in human movement was still present.

For example, I would find a rock to sit on and I would watch people as they walked by. At other times, I used to walk along the beach myself. I would follow behind people, observing their body alignment as they walked, and then I would look at the footprints they made in the sand to see how their weight was distributed as they moved. I soon learned to find the correlation between the two. You can learn a lot about people simply by watching how they carry themselves.

Try people-watching sometime. It can be amusing, and you may find that it is rather amazing as well. Perhaps it might even make you stop and think about your own alignment and the way you move. If someone were watching you, what would they see? What kind of stories does your own walk tell about you?

#6 LESSONS FROM BABIES

Have you ever watched a baby? Brand new human beings are always in motion. Watch the big movements of the baby, forever kicking his legs, rolling over and over, or scooting across the floor. Watch the small movements of a baby calming herself to sleep, or the even smaller movements of a sleeping baby, as he breathes with the whole diaphragm, lifting and expanding the rib cage up to the outer rotation of the arms before he exhales. Why then do we freeze, stiffen, and reduce our own possibilities for movement as we go through life?

#7 CHILDREN MIRROR PARENTS

Have you ever watched a mother and daughter walking together in the mall, a father and son walking into a restaurant to find a seat, or any other combination of family members, for that matter? When you watch children, you will usually find a mirror, a duplication of the parents' movement patterns. For generations, parents have unknowingly passed their own movement idiosyncracies on to their children. A child's internal temperament, rhythm, swing of the hips, posture, use or misuse of the swing of the arms and the shoulders, back rotation, shift of weight on the legs—all seem to have been unconsciously learned from the parent since infancy.

It would appear that human beings have forsaken many of their natural instincts for movement somewhere along the way. And still, with all the intelligence mankind has gained, we have to learn to sit, walk, and speak by trial and error and by watching our models.

#8 RECHANNELING MOVEMENT PATHS

I have a friend who once worked as a massage therapist. Then, while on vacation, she had a tobogganing accident and broke her tenth vertebra, right at her midback. The doctors who performed her surgery fused together the vertebras around the injured one.

Afterward, she asked them to prescribe physical therapy and machine work for her to strengthen her back, but their answer to her was not to waste her time; she would not walk again.

The community came to her side to help her. People from all sorts of body work professions volunteered their time and effort to work with her, believing it was possible to rechannel her movement paths along different routes of the body, in order to bypass the nerve damage. At the time that we worked with her, she was able to crawl and then stand.

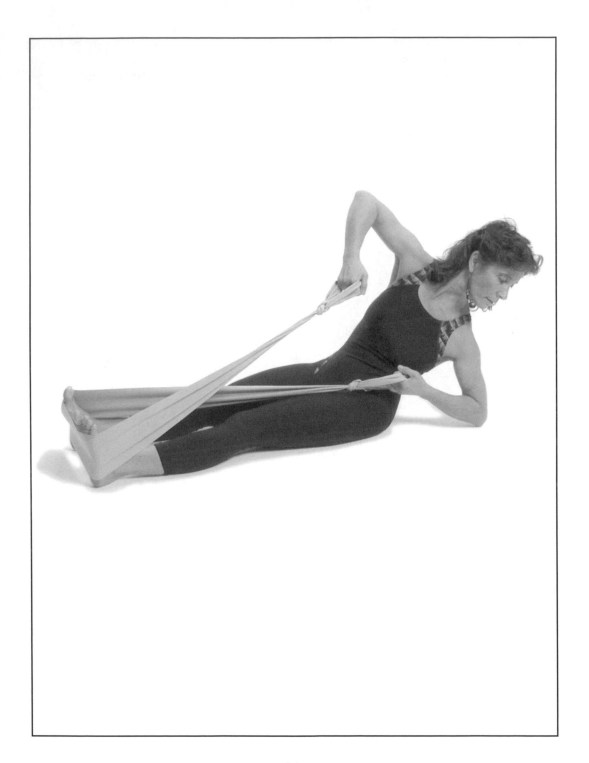

Chapter 2
Chapter Two: Exercises

PART 1: CENTER OF BODY

Our internal processes, provoked by present influences, or by forgotten, painful, previous experiences of the outside world, change our intentions to act as well as the way we act. You are as good as you wish; you are certainly more creative in imagining alternatives than you know. If you know "what" you are doing and even more important "how" you use your self to act, you will be able to do things the way you want. I believe that the world's most important advice, "Know thyself," was first said by one who learned to know oneself.

— Moshe Feldenkrais
The Elusive Obvious (1981: 70)

ABDOMINAL MUSCLES:

1. Rectus abdominis (2.1.1)
2. Obliques externus abdominis (2.1.2)
3. Obliques internus abdominis (2.1.3)
4. Transversus abdominis

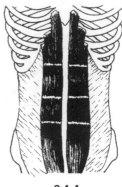

2.1.1

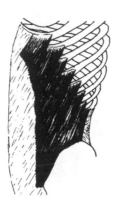

2.1.2

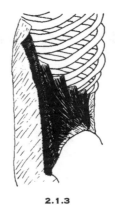

2.1.3

MUSCLES OF THE BACK:

1. Quadratus lumborum (2.1.4)
2. Splenius: capitas and cervicis (2.1.5)
3. Trapezius (2.1.5)

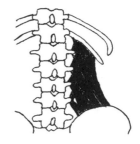

2.1.4

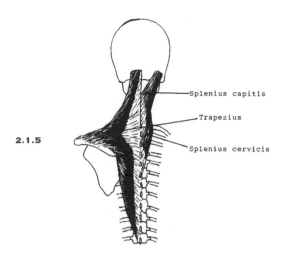

2.1.5

- Splenius capitis
- Trapezius
- Splenius cervicis

4. Transversospinalis

    A. Semispinalis: (cervicis and thoracis) (layer 1) (2.1.6)

    B. Multifidi (layer 2) (2.1.6)

    C. Rotators (layer 3) (2.1.7)

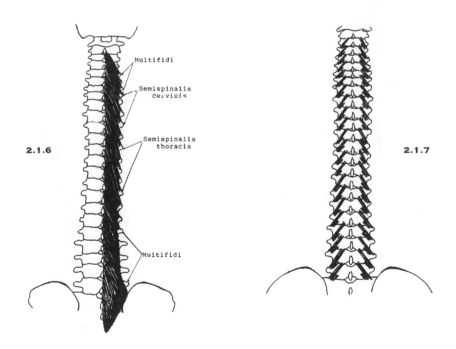

2.1.6

- Multifidi
- Semispinalis cervicis
- Semispinalis thoracis
- Multifidi

2.1.7

5. Erector spinae

   A. Spinalis

   B. Longissimus (capitas, cervicis, and dorsi) (2.1.8)

   C. Iliocostalis (cervicis, dorsi, and lumbo-rum) (2.1.8)

6. Interspinalis (tiny muscles deep to the overlying muscles)

7. Intertransversarii (tiny muscles deep to the overlying muscles)

8. Levator scapulae (2.1.9)

9. Rhomboid (major and minor) (2.1.9)

10. Latissimus dorsi (2.1.9)

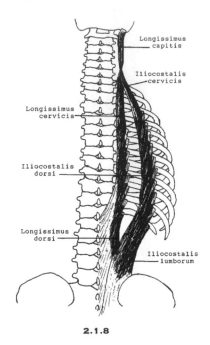

2.1.8

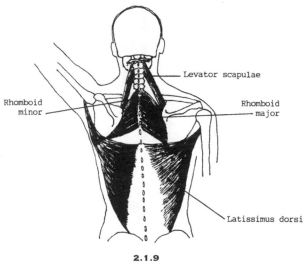

2.1.9

HIP FLEXOR:

Iliopsoas (2.1.10)

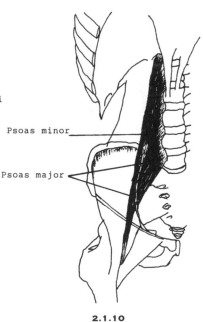

2.1.10

I. ABDOMINALS: THE ICE CREAM SCOOPER

POSITION: Sit on the floor on your sitting bones with your legs in front of you at a 90° angle. Flex your feet so that your toes point toward the ceiling. (2.1.11)

BAND: Place the center of the band on the soles of the feet, across the center of the foot (metatarsals). Cross each side of the band in front of the shins and hold in hands at a point on the band that will provide you with the appropriate amount of resistance.

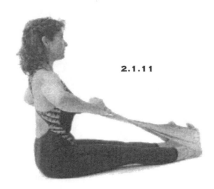

2.1.11

NOTE:

1. If your feet tend to turn in or out, wrap the band once around the feet so the band comes from the outside of each foot. Then cross the band in front of the shins.

2. The knees are softened slightly to prevent hyperextension. If you feel that using straight legs is too hard, you may place a towel, small pillow, or other support underneath them.

3. Arms are lifted and turned in so that the shoulders are pressed down. Think of the back widening, so that the latissimus dorsi muscle is being used throughout the exercise.

   • Be sure you are sitting on your sitting bones and not your lower back.

NOTE: You may do the exercise with bent legs/feet flat on the floor first.

EXERCISE:

1. BASIC—TAILBONE INITIATES LAST MOVE

   a. Exhale as you slowly lower your torso back toward the floor against the resistance of the band. (2.1.12)

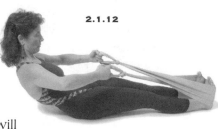

2.1.12

   • The curve of the spine will initiate from the spine's base and, in turn, will affect each successive vertebra.

   • Your neck will be last to curve, but it will not begin to curve until it is inevitable.

   • As you tilt your pelvis, imagine you are scooping out the contents of your abdomen, toward your spine and up toward your ribs.

b. Continue the scooping motion all the way down until your shoulders reach the floor.

   • Only go as low as you can without lifting your feet or falling. (2.1.13)

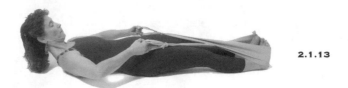

2.1.13

c. Without resting your weight on the floor, slowly return to the starting position by reversing the curving order of the vertebrae, starting with your head.

   • Use the same scooping sensation, and breath evenly.

   • Keep your elbows open and wide.

d. Once your head is directly in line over your tailbone—in a "C" shape—start to straighten your back with the movement initiating from the tailbone and continuing like a wave through each vertebra of the spine up to the head

2. BASIC—HEAD INITIATES LAST MOVE

   a. Repeat BASIC—TAILBONE INITIATES LAST MOVE starting on the previous page except straighten the spine by initiating the move ment with the head.

3. BASIC—CENTER OF BODY INITIATES LAST MOVE

   a. Repeat BASIC—TAILBONE INITIATES LAST MOVE starting on the previous page, except initiate the straightening of the spine from the center of your back instead of from the tailbone or head.

   • Both the head and tailbone will arrive at their final positions at the same time.

4. ADVANCED—WITH ONE HAND HOLDING

   a. Repeat #1–3, directly above, while holding both ends of the band in one hand.

   • Hold the other arm out to the side.

   • Be sure to keep both sides of the body equal or "square" as you do these exercises.

   b. Repeat, holding the band in the other hand.

II. ABDOMINALS: ROTATION

POSITION: Sit with your legs in front of you as in EXERCISE I: THE ICE CREAM SCOOPER. (2.1.14)

BAND: As in EXERCISE I: THE ICE CREAM SCOOPER, place the center of band on the soles of the feet, across the center of the foot (metatarsals). Cross each side of the band in front of the shins and hold in both hands at a point on the band that will provide you with the appropriate amount of resistance.

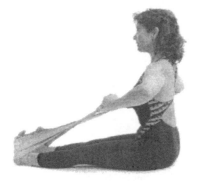

2.1.14

EXERCISES:

1. BASIC WITH STABLE HIPS AND FIXATED LEGS

   a. Pull your L elbow away from the R elbow as the back rotates to the L side. (2.1.15)

   • Your spine should be straight and as high as possible without the shoulders lifting or shrugging.

   • When you are rotated as far as you can, turn your head from side to side.

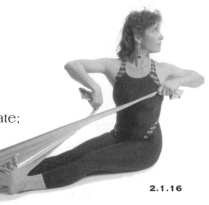

2.1.15

NOTE: Be sure you are sitting directly on top of the sitting bones (your ischial tuberosities), and the spine rotates on top of the fixed pelvis. This will isolate the rotation muscle along your spine in order to rotate to each side.

   b. Return to center, starting position.

   c. Repeat on second side.

2. BASIC WITH ROTATING HIPS

   a. Repeat #1, directly above.

   • As you rotate to the L side this time, the pelvis will also be allowed to rotate; the L leg will shorten into the hip socket while the R leg seems to lengthen and grow longer (without bending at the knee). (2.1.16)

2.1.16

   b. Return to center, starting position.

   c. Repeat on second side.

3. ADVANCED (not on the video)

   a. Repeat EXERCISES 1 and 2: BASIC with
      your legs a little wider than hips-width
      apart. (2.1.17)

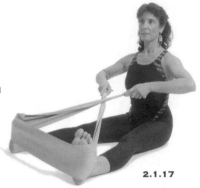

2.1.17

III. ABDOMINAL COMBINATION

   The following directions are for the same starting position
of EXERCISES I and II on pages 43 and 45.

   POSITION: Sit on the floor on your sitting bones with
your legs in front of you at a 90° angle. Flex your feet so
that your toes point toward the ceiling. (2.1.18)

   BAND: Place the center of band on the soles
of the feet, across the metatarsals. Cross each
side of the band in front of the shins and hold
in the opposite hand at a point on the band
that will provide you with the appropriate
amount of resistance. Start with the R hand on top.

2.1.18

   EXERCISES: (combination of EXERCISES I and II)

1. BASIC

   a. Curve the spine to lower your torso to the floor, initiating the move-
      ment from the base of the spine and scooping the
      abdomen as in EXERCISE I. At the same time, rotate
      the hip and back to the L side as in EXERCISE II.

      • Keep your arms and elbows at the same
        distance and relationship from the body
        as you move.

      • End up with your L elbow on
        the floor diagonally behind
        you, and your R elbow
        pointing 180° (straight line)
        from it in the air. (2.1.19)

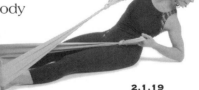

2.1.19

b. Return to the starting position by reversing the movement.

c. Change the band so that the band end in your L hand is on top. Repeat on the second side, starting with scooping and rotating to the right.

2. ADVANCED: SCOOP, ROTATE, EXTEND ARM

a. Repeat EXERCISE 1: BASIC, directly above, rolling the spine down to the floor, "scooping out" your abdomen, and rotating to the L. At the same time, extend the R arm, forearm, and hand to a straightened position 180° from the opposite elbow. (2.1.20)

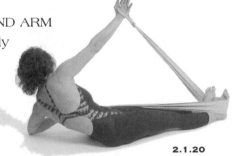

2.1.20

b. Repeat on the second side, changing the band so that the L hand in on top.

3. ADVANCED: ONE HAND, TWO FEET

a. Hold both loops in the L hand (the side to which you rotate), and repeat EXERCISE 2, directly above.

• Point the L elbow diagonally behind you as the spine lengthens down to the floor.

• Hold the R arm out to the side of the body, in a straight line from the L elbow through the R hand. (2.1.21)

b. Repeat on the right side, being sure to change the loops to the R hand.

4. ADVANCED: ONE FOOT, ONE HAND HOLDS (not on video)

STARTING POSITION: Wrap both loops around the both feet and hold the center of the band with your L hand, so your body acts in opposition. Contract your abdominals inward toward your spine as you rotate to the L side.

2.1.21

a. Repeat all of EXERCISE 2 in this new position.

IV. ILIOPSOAS STRETCH

POSITION: Place each end of the band on each foot and lie on your back with the legs about hips-width apart. Bend both knees and point them up toward the ceiling. Place the soles of the feet flat on the floor near your hips.

- Be sure to keep the natural curve in your back with your hips "neutral". The waist will neither push into the floor (flattening the back) nor pull away from the floor (over-arching the spine).

BAND:

1. With a loop on each foot, lay the band along the floor beside the legs.
2. With both hands, grasp the band from underneath at its center.
3. Pull the band to your waist.
   - If you want a stronger stretch, place it underneath the elbows and across the upper arm, pulling it to your chest.

EXERCISE:

1. SIMPLE: ONE FOOT
   a. As you exhale, flex the L foot and slowly straighten the L leg by sliding the heel along the floor.
      - Think of lengthening the leg out from the heel.
      - Feel the back of the leg stretching.
      - Use the flattened abdominal muscles to support the back.
   b. As you exhale, slowly draw the L foot back in as you bend the L leg.
   c. Repeat on the second side.

2. SIMPLE: TWO FEET

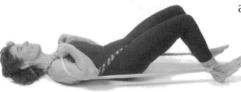

2.1.22

   a. As you exhale, flex both feet and slowly straighten the legs by sliding the heels along the floor. (2.1.22)
      - Hold the lower back close to the floor and do not release it throughout the whole exercise. Do not push it into the floor either.
      - Reach out with the feet even farther.

b. As you exhale, slowly draw the feet back in as you bend the legs.

3. VARIATION

   a. After fully extending the legs, simultaneously raise the head and legs a few inches from the floor. Exhale the whole time. (2.1.23)

   b. After taking a brief breath, exhale as you reverse these movements to return to the starting position.

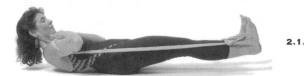

2.1.23

4. SIMPLE: ON YOUR SIDE

STARTING POSITION: Lie on your L side with knees bent.

BAND: Attach the band to the R flexed foot—the top foot. Run it behind your back and hold it with both hands behind your head.

   • Your arms will be bent, elbows near the sides of your head.

   a. Lengthen the R leg (top leg) from the heel as you did in the SIMPLE version.

   b. Once your leg is straight, extend the lengthening as you reach your leg behind you.

      • Only try this if you feel you can.

      • Don't go into an arc. Remember that the abdominals support the back.

   c. Exhale as you retrace your leg's path.

   d. Turn to the other side, change the band, and repeat parts a.–c.

V. LEG STRETCH

POSITION: Sit on your sitting bones.

BAND: You have your choice in band placement.

1. *Easier:* Place one loop on each foot and hold the band in both hands, about shoulder width apart and in front of your ribs, as you see in the photo. Bend the L knee and keep the R leg straight. (2.1.24)

2.1.24

2. *More difficult:* Place the loops of the band on the sole of the L foot. Bend both knees. Place the band on each side of the L leg and hold it in each hand. (on video)

EXERCISE:

1. SIMPLE: PARALLEL

    a. By lengthening out from the heel, extend your L leg and straighten your leg along the floor.

       • Do not allow the knee joint to hyperextend backward. That is, always bring the lower leg toward the thigh rather than letting the knee go back and toward the floor.

    b. Slowly bend your knee again.

    c. Repeat, lengthening your leg a little higher each time (4–5 repetitions), i.e., each bend and extension will be a little higher off the floor. (2.1.25 and 2.1.26)

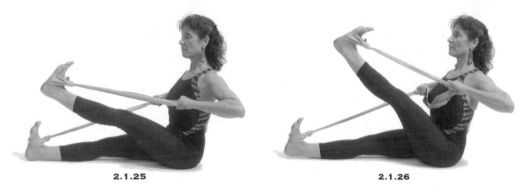

2.1.25   2.1.26

      • Keep your back erect.

      • Keep your elbows wide and lifted.

    d. After the highest extension, simply lower the straight leg to the floor and bend the knee to return to the starting position.

    e. Repeat on the second side.

2. SIMPLE: TURNED OUT

STARTING POSITION: Turn your working bent leg out at the hip socket.

    a. Repeat #1 SIMPLE: PARALLEL in this position.

3. SIMPLE: TURNED IN

STARTING POSITION: Turn your bent leg in at the hip socket so that your L foot and knee face your R leg.

    a. Repeat #1 SIMPLE: PARALLEL in this position.

4. Repeat all exercises on the second side.

VI. SPINAL CHAIN

POSITION: Stand with your legs parallel to one another. Place your arms overhead a little wider than shoulder width apart. (2.1.27)

BAND: Hold the band in both hands.

EXERCISE:

1. SIMPLE

    a. Rolling down: Slowly curve and roll the spine from the head down to the tailbone. At the same time, open the arms to the sides, while slowly descending (gravitating) with the torso toward the floor. (2.1.28)

- The band will lie across the shoulder blades or slightly underneath them.
- The abdominal muscles contract toward the spine, the chin is dropped down toward the chest, and the knees bend softly.

    b. Rolling Up: Reaching the lowest point of your back extension (when you are the most bent forward), keep your arms lengthened loosely down toward the floor. (2.1.29) Rise as your torso contracts and slowly pulls back up toward the ceiling.

- Remember to start the movement in your pelvis with your abdominals, and keep the neck and head loose.

    c. Once the arms reach shoulder height, rotate the arms slowly and extend them to overhead (the starting position).

- Remember to keep the shoulder blades (scapulae) depressed.

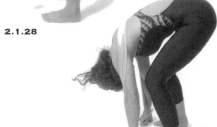

2.1.29

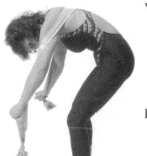

2.1.28

2.1.27

2. VARIATION: HUG (not on video)

    a. Rolling down: As above, curve and roll the spine from the head down to the tailbone.

    b. On the way down, once you contract the abdominal muscles, stay in the contraction and cross your arms in front of your chest as if you were hugging yourself. (2.1.30)

    c. Return slowly by lifting the arms and back up at the same time. (See EXERCISE 1-b, Rolling Up, above for details on how to roll up.)

    d. Repeat this Variation once with the R arm in front on the "hug," and once with the L arm in front.

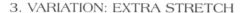

2.1.30

3. VARIATION: EXTRA STRETCH

    a. Roll down as described above.

    b. While you are down, place one loop on each foot so you are standing on them.

    c. Place the elbows against the band within the width of the band.

    d. Exhale as you pull yourself upward while drawing your shoulder blades down.

    e. Repeat c. and d.

    f. Remove the loops from your feet and stand up.

Lessons from Life

#1 A GOOD END FOR WARM-UP

When I was a dance student in college, my body was cold and stiff early in the morning. One of my favorite exercises to do at the *end* of my warm-up was to get into the yoga plow position. First, lie on your back on the floor. Bring your legs up and over your head, letting your pelvis come up as well, until your toes touch the floor above your head. The stretching sensation will expand and crawl up and down your spine. When I do this, I feel as though I can trace the nervous system from my spinal column through the rest of my body, just like the diagrams you see in physiology books. (Be sure not to put all your weight on the neck vertebrae but keep it along the whole torso.)

#2 FINDING YOUR WAY

There are no hard rules. Everyone has his or her own individual body language and develops his or her own inner logic. Maybe this is the reason there are so many techniques for "body work" and approaches to reach mind-body and soul. If none really appeals to help you, then it is the time to look inside yourself and create your own. Listen to your body's messages and try to recognize how to interpret them to your best ability. The key to your own body language is always somewhere inside yourself.

#3 FLEXIBILITY OF MIND AND BODY

I have a friend with whom I've worked since 1984. She lived until she was over seventy years old. When she was fourteen, she had severe pains that prevented her from walking. The doctor found it to be degeneration of the joint between the pelvis and the leg. He fused the joint into an angle, causing the lower back to act as a joint instead. Years later, while she was in her forties, her back gave out. The doctors had to reset the fused joint into a different angle. This wonderful woman never lost her smile. She always continued her community work and her concern for others. Most of all, in spite of the pain and discomfort of her movement limitation, she learned new ways to cope, so she could move and dance with grace for the remainder of her life. Thank you, Jackie Jacobs, I have learned a lot from you.

#4 TO THINK ABOUT

Did you ever stop to think that if you warm up your body for physical activity by starting at the head and progressing down to your feet, different energy results than if you start at your feet and work your way up to your head?

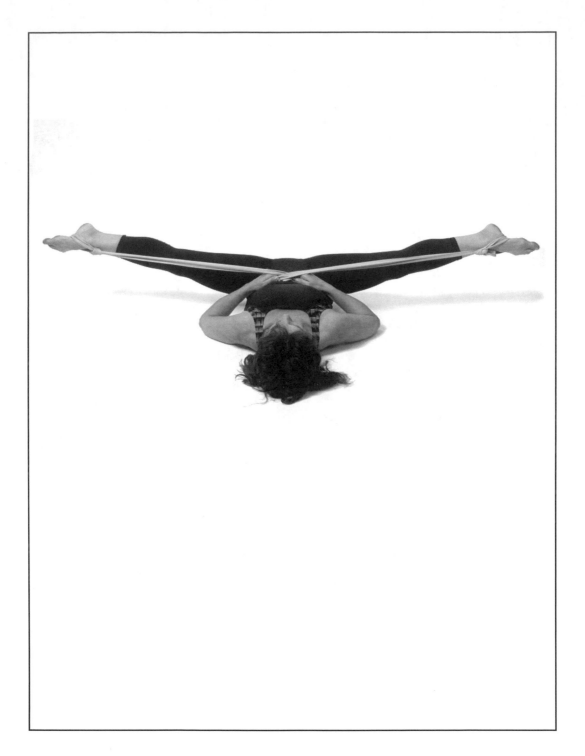

Chapter 2

Chapter Two: Exercises

PART 2: LOWER BODY

To be alive, to know life, is to breathe. To breathe is to move, to move is to change. Movement is fundamental to life.

— Diane Mariechild
The Inner Dance (1987: Introduction)

THE MAIN MUSCLE GROUPS USED IN PART 2

MUSCLES FOR HIP ADDUCTION:

1. Pectineus (2.2.1)
2. Gracilis (2.2.1)
3. Adductor longus (2.2.1)
4. Adductor brevis (2.2.1)
5. Adductor magnus (2.2.1)

MUSCLES FOR HIP ABDUCTION

1. Tensor fasciae latae (2.2.3)
2. Gluteus medius (2.2.2)
3. Gluteus minimus (2.2.2)
4. The six deep rotators
   A. Piriformis
   B. Superior gemellus (2.2.2)
   C. Obturator internus (2.2.2)
   D. Inferior gemellus (2.2.2)
   E. Obturator externus (2.2.2)
   F. Quadratus femoris (2.2.2)

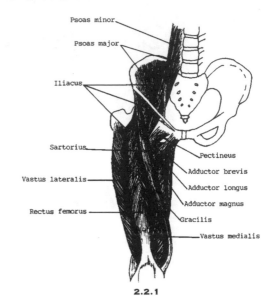

2.2.1

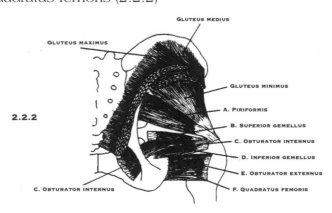

2.2.2

MUSCLE GROUP OF THE POSTERIOR THIGH: HAMSTRING

1. Biceps femoris (2.2.3)
2. Semitendinosus (2.2.3)
3. Semimembranosus (2.2.3)

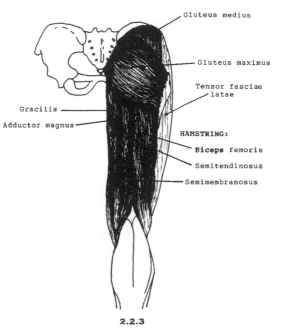

MUSCLE GROUP OF THE ANTERIOR THIGH: QUADRICEPS

1. Rectus femoris (2.2.1)
2. Vastus lateralis (2.2.1)
3. Vastus medialis (2.2.1)
4. Vastus intermedius

MUSCLES FOR INWARD ROTATION OF THE HIP

1. Tensor fasciae latae (2.2.3 and 2.2.4)
2. Gluteus minimus (in femur abduction) (2.2.4)
3. Semitendinosus (2.2.3)
4. Gracilis (2.2.3)

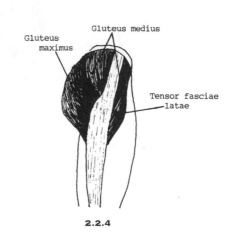

MUSCLES FOR OUTWARD ROTATION OF THE HIP

1. Gluteus medius (in hip abduction) (2.2.5)
2. Gluteus maximus (2.2.5)
3. The six deep lateral rotator muscles
   A. Piriformis
   B. Superior gemellus (2.2.5)
   C. Obturator internus (2.2.5)
   D. Inferior gemellus (2.2.5)
   E. Obturator externus (2.2.5)
   F. Quadratus femoris (2.2.5)
4. Iliopsoas (in thigh flexion): psoas minor and major (2.2.1)
5. Sartorius (in thigh flexion) (2.2.1)
6. Biceps femoris (2.2.3)
7. Adductor brevis (in hip adduction) (2.2.1)
8. Adductor magnus (in hip adduction) (2.2.1)

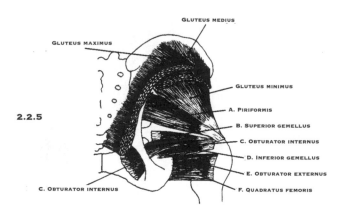

MUSCLE FOR HIP AND KNEE FLEXION

Sartorius (2.2.1)

MUSCLE FOR KNEE FLEXION

Popliteus (2.2.6)

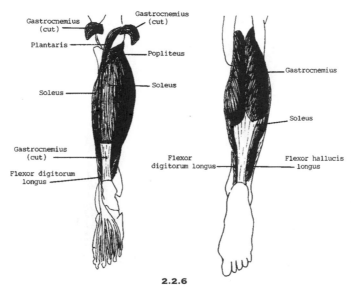

2.2.6

MUSCLES OF THE CALF AND FOOT

1. Plantar flexors

2. Gastrocnemius (2.2.6)

3. Flexor digitorum longus (2.2.6)

4. Flexor hallucis longus (2.2.6)

5. Peroneus longus (2.2.7)

6. Peroneus brevis

7. Plantaris (2.2.6)

8. Soleus (2.2.6)

9. Tibialis posterior

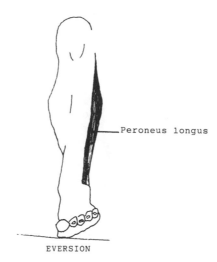

EVERSION

2.2.7

MUSCLES FOR DORSI FLEXION OF THE FOOT

1. Extensor digitorum longus (2.2.8)
2. Extensor hallucis longus (2.2.9)
3. Tibialis anterior (2.2.9)

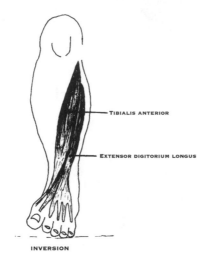

INVERSION

2.2.8

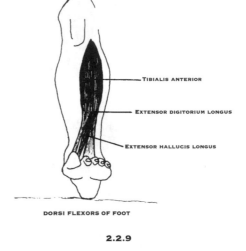

DORSI FLEXORS OF FOOT

2.2.9

I. ANTIGRAVITY LEG WORK

POSITION: Lie on your back with both legs held at a 90°
angle up in the air. Flex the feet as if you were standing on
the ceiling. (2.2.10)

- By keeping the legs directly above the hip, you will
  work the leg extensors, especially those behind the
  knees.

NOTE: Sensing where 90° is in this position
may be difficult; most people tend to have their
legs leaning too far forward or backward. Therefore, it would be a good idea to do exercises in this
position with a mirror nearby, or better yet, with the legs up
against a wall. If you can't bring the legs to 90°, bend your knees slightly
and raise the legs so the feet are over the pelvis.

2.2.10

BAND:

1. Place the ends of the band on both feet.
2. Cross the band in front of the shins, and
3. Hold it in your hands at a point on the band that will provide you with
   the appropriate amount of resistance.
4. Place your elbows and upper arms on the floor beside you.
   - Your back will be wide and open.
5. Be sure that you are in the starting position described above.

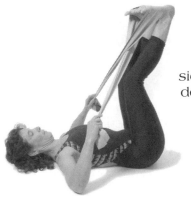

2.2.11

EXERCISE:

1. SIMPLE

STARTING POSITION: Legs are parallel with the
sides of the feet together, in the starting position
described above.

a. Slowly bend the knees, creating an imaginary straight line between your heels and
   tailbone. (2.2.11)

- Do not let your upper legs lean toward
  your face. They remain at 90°.

- Be sure your spine remains in a straight
  line from head to tailbone.

- Be sure your pelvis does not tilt as the
  knees bend.

61

b. Keeping the feet flexed, push the heels upward to slowly move the knees toward straight.

- The center of the kneecaps should be on an imaginary line between your second and third toes.
- You should feel a stretch from the heels to the tailbone in opposite directions—heels to the ceiling, tailbone to the floor.
- Make sure you do not push your knees backward (i.e., do not hyperextend your knees).

2. TURN IN AND TURN OUT

a. Rotate out your whole leg so the heels are touching and the toes are away from them. (2.2.12)

b. Rotate in your whole leg to return to parallel.

- This action takes place in the hip socket.
- Do not hyperextend your knees. If you do, you will create a space between your heels.

3. THE DIAMOND

STARTING POSITION: Keeping your heels together, rotate your legs outward from the hip socket into a ballet 1st position. (2.2.13)

- Do not let your legs turn out more at your feet than at your hip joints.

a. Starting in this turned-out first position, repeat #1: SIMPLE, above— bending and straightening your legs.

- As you bend your knees, do not let your feet turn out more than your knees or hips.

NOTE: Rest between sections by turning legs to parallel and bending the knees.

4. DIAGONAL ARROW:

STARTING POSITION: Starting in 1st position, as in #3: DIAMOND, above, bend the knees in a plié. (2.2.13)

- Be sure you don't bend your knees too much. Really keep a diamond shape that is longer than it is wide.

2.2.13

62

a. Without moving the thigh, straighten the R leg in a diagonal to the R side to complete the line of the thigh. (2.2.14)

   • Both R and L feet remain flexed.

b. Bend the R knee to return to 1st position diamond shape.

c. Do the same with your L leg.

5. DOUBLE DIAGONAL ARROW

STARTING POSITION: Starting in 1st position, as in #3: DIAMOND, above, bend the knees in a plié.

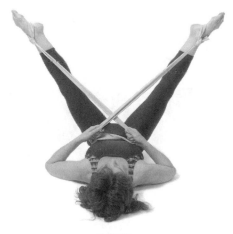

2.2.14

a. Similar to #4 DIAGONAL ARROW, straighten both legs diagonally to complete the lines of the thighs at the same time.

b. Bend the knees to return to 1st position diamond shape.

c. Straighten both legs with flexed feet reaching to the ceiling.

d. Repeat a. and b. above with knees bent a little deeper so knees are father apart and legs straighten wider.

e. Repeat again with legs bent more to your maximum.

NOTE: You may point the feet when you open the legs. (2.2.15)

2.2.15

6. SCISSORS

STARTING POSITION: Turned out legs—at 90°—are crossed one in front of the other (in a ballet fifth position) in the air or against a wall. Feet remain flexed.

    a. Use a wide scissors kick to open the legs to second position. (2.2.16)

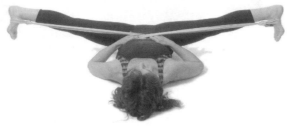

2.2.16

    b. Return to fifth position again, alternating which foot is in front each time.

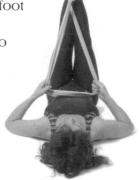

- Alternate the position of the feet from flexed to pointed. (2.2.17 and 2.2.18)

- Begin slowly and increase the speed (tempo) with control.

- Make sure the abdominals remain in use. Do not allow the lower back to move and shift with the leg movement.

2.2.17

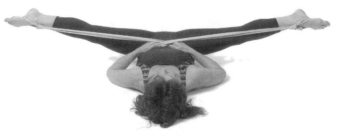

2.2.18

7. PARALLEL SIMPLE

STARTING POSITION: Start with your legs in a parallel second position, a little wider than hip-width apart.

- a. Bend and straighten one leg.
    - Straighten by lengthening out from the heels.
- b. Bend and straighten the other leg.
- c. Bend and straighten both legs. (2.2.19)
- d. Bend both legs, bring them together, and lengthen (straighten) them up to the ceiling.
- e. Bend and open wide to do the opening and closing as in #6 SCISSORS, above. (2.2.19)
- f. After several repetitions of the Scissors, bend you knees closer to your chest and rest.

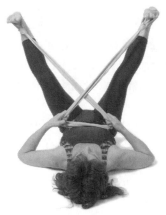

2.2.19

II. ADVANCED ANTIGRAVITY LEGWORK

POSITION: Lie on your back, legs at a 90° angle in the air (or against a wall). Legs should be rotated outward, in the hip joint, to a ballet first position.

BAND: The band should be in the same position as in EXERCISE I: ANTIGRAVITY LEGWORK on page 61 (2.2.20)

EXERCISE:

1. SIMPLE (not on the video):

    a. Instead of I. ANTIGRAVITY LEGWORK, #5 SCISSORS open the legs into a wide second position.

        • Flexed toes should face the floor. (2.2.21)

        • Do not tilt the pelvis off of the floor.

    b. Bend your knees, turning your legs out even more.

    c. Straighten your legs by lengthening out from the pelvis through the heels.

        • You will probably feel a stretch behind the knee.

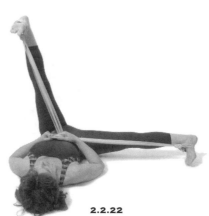

2.2.20

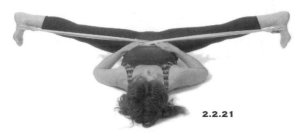

2.2.21

    d. Repeat, bending your knees in the wide position as many times as in your program.

    e. Lift both legs slowly as you return to the starting position.

2. SINGLE LEG

    a. Lower one leg to the floor directly to the side, keeping the other leg up in the air (2.2.22); then return to the starting position.

2.2.22

- Both sides of the pelvis stay stable and on the floor.
- Flex or point the feet as desired.

b. Repeat with the second leg.

c. Repeat, lowering one leg directly in front of you (2.2.23); then return.

- The working leg will lower to be in line with your spine.
- Remember not to arch your lower back as the leg lowers.

d. Repeat with the second leg, changing the crossing of the band so that the side connected to the working foot is underneath the other side's band.

NOTE: You will be unable to complete this exercise if your legs are against a wall. You will need to move away from the wall.

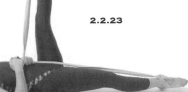

2.2.23

III. LYING ON ONE SIDE

POSITION:

a. Lie on the R side of your body.

b. Bend the bottom (R) leg, and flex the toes, so they can be braced against the floor for support.

c. Extend the top (L) leg parallel to the floor.

- The bottom leg's knee, hip, and shoulder should remain in one line.
- Support your body with your top (L) hand in front of your stomach, so you do not roll forward or backward.
- Try to keep the lower ribs closed and slightly lifted off the floor. (The waist will always be slightly lifted off the floor.) (2.2.24)

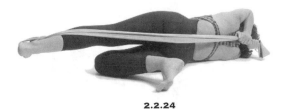

2.2.24

- To be sure your spine remains straight, be especially careful that your ribs do not release when you execute a movement to the back while in this position. Instead, both sides of the ribs should be aligned with one side directly on top of the other.

BAND: Attach one end of the band to the top foot. Then, stretch the band along the side of the body and behind the back. Hold the band behind your neck with both hands, at a point on the band that is appropriate to you.

NOTE: If this position is uncomfortable for you, you may hold the band by spreading it over your top shoulder and stabilizing it with the top hand.

EXERCISE:

1. SIMPLE LENGTHENING

STARTING POSITION: Flex your top foot parallel to the floor, and no more than three inches off the floor. (2.2.24)
   a. Without using a large movement, lengthen your top leg out of the hip socket.
      - The knee stays straight.
   b. Then, shorten the leg back into the hip socket.
      - Work with the pelvis moving with the leg.
      - Make sure the hip muscles and the abdominals initiate the movement.
   c. Repeat a. and b. several times.

2. ROTATION INWARD AND OUTWARD, WITH LOW LEG
   a. Rotate the top leg in, turning your toes and the top knee down toward the floor. (This works the tensor fasciae latae.) (2.2.25)

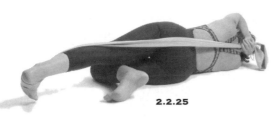

2.2.25

- Make sure the hip muscles and the abdominals initiate the movement.
   b. Return the entire leg and pelvis to the starting parallel position. (2.2.24)

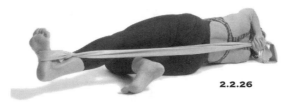

2.2.26

c. Continue to turn out the entire leg and pelvis. (2.2.26)

- Allow your hip to roll forward and return with the leg movement in a. and b.

d. After several repetitions fixate the hip to isolate the leg, doing the work within the hip socket. That is, the hip will not be allowed to roll forward and return with the leg movement.

3. ROTATION INWARD AND OUTWARD, WITH LEG HIGHER (not on video)

STARTING POSITION: Keeping the knee of the top leg forward (leg parallel), lift your leg until it is slightly higher than the hip.

a. At that height, rotate the leg in and out.

NOTE: Roll the hip at first, with the leg movement. Then, isolate the movement of the leg from the hip.

4. PARALLEL PULSING

STARTING POSITION: Keeping the top leg parallel (with the knee facing forward), lift your leg until it is slightly higher than the hips, as in #3: ROTATION INWARD AND OUTWARD, WITH LEG HIGHER directly above. (2.2.27)

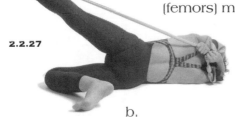

2.2.27

NOTE: The parallel position of the top leg with toes and knee forward will limit the height the leg can rise. (The thigh bones (femors) meet the hip bone (ilium).)

a. With the foot flexed, once you reach the maximum height to the side, do small bounces, gently raising and lowering the leg in order to strengthen the abductors. (not on video)

Repeat this exercise with the foot

b. pointed. (not on video)

5. LEG STRETCH SIDE

STARTING POSITION

- Keeping your body alignment, turn your top leg out, so knee faces the ceiling. (2.2.28)
- Lift the top leg up to the side as far as you can, fixating the bottom leg to the floor. (2.2.29)
- Shorten the band to achieve the resistance that is right or you.

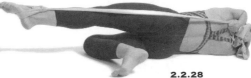

2.2.28

- The foot is flexed or pointed, depending on your need that day.

69

a. Bend the knee.

b. Lengthen the leg by bringing the lower part of the leg up to the line of the thigh.

c. Repeat several times.

- Each time you bend the leg, you can increase the bend to increase the stretch of the leg as it straightens to meet the line of the thigh (which will be closer to your torso).

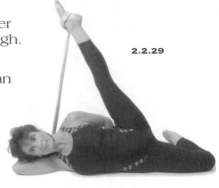

2.2.29

d. After several repetitions, lengthen the leg toward the bottom leg.

- Be sure the working leg lengthens out of its hip socket.

6. LEG LIFTS SIDE

STARTING POSITION: Use the same starting position as #5: LEG STRETCH SIDE. (2.2.28) Then lower the top leg back down to the bent bottom leg.

a. With your top foot flexed, lift and lower the top leg as you did to get into position. (not on video)

b. Repeat this exercise with the top foot pointed.

7. REST AND REPEAT ON THE SECOND SIDE

a. Rest by rolling onto your back and bend your legs to hug your knees.

b. While you rest, change the band to the other foot.

c. Do parts #1–6 on the second side.

8. LEG LIFTS FRONT

STARTING POSITION: Starting with the top leg down, lift it to in front of the body.

a. Keeping the bottom leg stable, lengthen your parallel top leg to your maximum extension in front of you. (2.2.30)

b. "Shorten" the leg into the hip as you return to the starting position.

- Allow your hip to move forward and backward with the leg.

2.2.30

- Hold the band as before or stretch the band over your opposite shoulder on the ground. *Use the position which is more comfortable for you.*

9. LEG LIFT FRONT II (not on video)

STARTING POSITION: Lift the top leg directly in front of your body, keeping the foot about three inches off the floor. Shorten the band, if necessary, to achieve the resistance that is right for you. Then return the top leg down to the bent bottom leg.

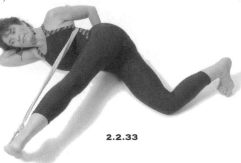

2.2.31

NOTE: Your flexibility (the length of your extensor muscles) determines how high you raise your leg in front of you. Be sure not to disturb your proper alignment. Your bottom knee, hip, and shoulder should be in one line.

a. With the leg in parallel position and the foot flexed, lift the top leg directly in front of your body, keeping the foot at about three inches off the floor, and return it to the bottom leg.

b. Repeat the leg lift front with your top foot pointed. (2.2.31)

c. Repeat the leg lift front with the leg rotated outward (turned out)—once with the foot flexed, then with the foot pointed. (2.2.32)

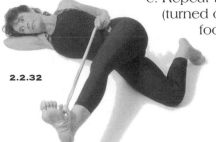

2.2.32

d. Repeat the leg lift front with the leg rotated inward (turned in) beyond parallel. Toes will be toward the floor, rotated inward as far as possible (everted), once with the foot flexed, and then pointed. (2.2.33)

10. LEG MOVES BEHIND YOU (not on video)

STARTING POSITION: Keeping the bottom leg stable, lift your top leg toward the ceiling, with leg turned out and the foot flexed. Shorten the band. Bend this leg slightly and bring the thigh behind your body to create an arched shape.

2.2.33

- The toes of the bottom leg are curled under for support.
- This will feel as if someone had pulled your foot.
- Keep the shape of the leg, but open the angle of the knee wider.
- This is like a ballet attitude. (2.2.34)

a. Moving toward and away from the floor (behind your bottom leg) lower and lift the entire leg as a single unit to maintain the relationship of the thigh to the lower leg.

11. STRAIGHT LEG BEHIND

STARTING POSITION: Bend your knee of the top leg into an arched position as in the last exercise, #10: LEG MOVES BEHIND YOU. (2.2.34)

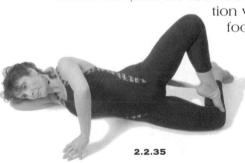

2.2.34

a. Straighten your leg directly behind you in a long, straight line by pushing outward from the heel.

• The lower part of your working leg will make one straight line with the upper leg.

b. Bend your leg slowly as you return to the starting position.

12. TURN IN/TURN OUT, LEG BEHIND

STARTING POSITION: Begin in the same attitude position as the last two exercises, #9: LEG MOVES BEHIND YOU and #11: STRAIGHT LEG BEHIND.

a. Swing your top leg gently from a position with the upper thigh turned out (and the foot touching the other knee) (2.2.35) to a position with the upper thigh turned in (and the foot in the air behind the body).

NOTE: Your thigh acts as an axis so be sure the thigh and knee remain in the same relationship to each other as you raise and lower your foot and lower leg. Always stay in control.

2.2.35

13. REST AND REPEAT ON THE SECOND SIDE

a. Turn the top, bent leg in and lower it on top of the bottom bent leg.

b. Roll onto your back with knees into your chest.

c. Change the band to the other foot.

d. Repeat #8–12 on the second side.

IV. THE HINGE: Hamstring Group

POSITION: Lie on the L side with your R, top leg straightened and your bottom leg bent at the knee as in EXERCISE III: LYING ON ONE SIDE.

- Be sure to keep the knee, hip, and shoulder in one line.

BAND: Attach one end of the band to the top foot. Stretch the band behind the back. Hold the band behind the neck with both hands. (2.2.36)

NOTE: If this position is too difficult for you, spread the center of the band over the upper shoulder and stabilize it with your upper hand.

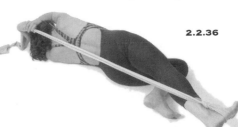

2.2.36

EXERCISE:

1. SIMPLE EXERCISE

  a. Bend the top leg to match the bottom leg and shorten the band. (2.2.37)

- Your lower working leg will move behind the body while your thigh remains in place, so the hamstrings will be worked.

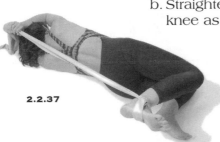

2.2.37

  b. Straighten your top leg at the knee, using the knee as a hinge.

- Be sure your leg stays parallel to the floor as you do this exercise.

  c. Repeat bending and straightening the top leg.

2. VARIATION

  a. Point the foot as you bend the leg.

  b. Flex the foot as you extend/lengthen the leg.

3. SECOND SIDE: Change the band to the L foot and repeat all parts on the second side.

73

V. POSTERIOR: THE JUNGLE CAT

POSITION: Place your body in the all-fours position on your hands and knees. Straighten your back to create a 90° angle from your arms to your torso, and from your thighs to your torso. (2.2.38)

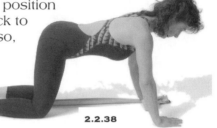

2.2.38

- Your abdominals should support your lower back by pulling in toward your spine and up toward your ribs.

BAND: Place one end of the band on your R foot. Stretch it between your legs, under your body, and hold the other end with your L hand.

NOTE: Advanced version: Place both ends of the band on your R foot. Stretch it between your legs, under your body, and hold the center of it with your L hand.

- The abdominals must remain working throughout the whole exercise. They pull in toward the spine and up toward the ribs to support your lower back.
- Keep your rib cage closed like an umbrella, and bend your elbows slightly.
- Your back is like a tabletop as you keep a straight line between your head and your tailbone.
- Do not allow your weight to shift to the opposite hand when working with the leg to the side. Keep your body centered.

EXERCISE:

1. SIMPLE

FLATBACK (not on video)

  a. Lengthen your R leg behind you by sliding the top of the toes and the top of your foot on the floor, stretching the top of the front of your thigh (quadriceps). (2.2.39)

2.2.39

  b. Return to the original position.

WITH ARCH

  a. Repeat #1: SIMPLE, above, arching your back as the leg is extended to the back, with the head and eyes going upward to continue the arch.

74

b. As the leg returns, either return to the starting position or curve the back and draw the head and pelvis toward each other.

  • This exercise works the head/tail relationship.

2. OFF THE FLOOR

a. Lengthen your R leg behind you by sliding it on the floor; then lift it to the height of your back as your upper body continues the arc. (2.2.40)

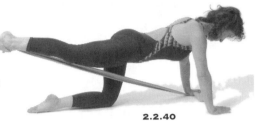

2.2.40

b. Return to the original position by reversing the movement.

NOTE: EXERCISES 1 and 2 work well as a warm-up.

3. EXTENDED FARTHER

SIMPLE

a. Slide the R leg back, as in #1: SIMPLE, above.

b. Continue to move it back even farther, as if someone were pulling it.

  • Your whole torso will move toward your extended foot and your arms will hinge at the shoulder.

  • The foot stays on the floor. (2.2.41)

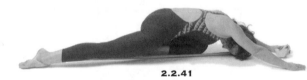

2.2.41

c. Return.

  • You will feel a strong shift of weight backward on your hands so allow the back to move with the leg and keep the elbows slightly bent.

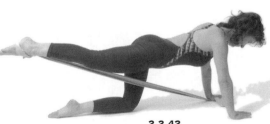

2.2.42

  • The chin comes closer to the chest as your weight pulls back, and your head becomes aligned with your spine as you return to all-fours.

NOTE: Variation: You may look up on a diagonal as you pull back away from all-fours.

75

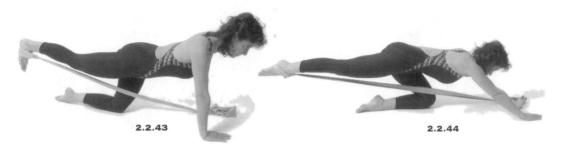

2.2.43   2.2.44

VARIATION (not on video):

  a. Begin as you did in #4: EXTENDED FARTHER, but extend the leg
     out and up as high as your back. (2.2.42, 2.2.43, 2.2.44, 2.2.45,
     and 2.2.46)

  b. Return to the starting position.

NOTE: Flex the foot as your leg moves outward to the back (2.2.43), and
point it as it returns. (2.2.44)

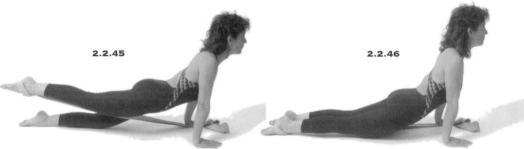

2.2.45   2.2.46

4. SIDE LEG REACHES

BEGINNING

  a. Slide the R foot on the floor behind you as in the #1: SIMPLE ver-
     sion of this exercise. (2.2.39)

  b. Straighten the knee as you slide it to the R side up to a
     comfortable extension. The big toe will remain
     on the floor. (2.2.47)

  c. Slide it behind you again, with the foot still on
     the floor.

  d. Return to the original all-fours position.

NOTE: This may be done with the
band beneath you, as in #1–3, or the band
can run across your back, over the L shoulder
and to the L hand on the floor.

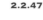

2.2.47

ADVANCED

a. Repeat #4 SIDE LEG REACHES,
above, with the leg at the height
of your back. (2.2.48)

• The leg is extended to the back,
rotates out in the socket as you
move it to the side, and returns
to parallel (knee faces down) as it moves
back again.

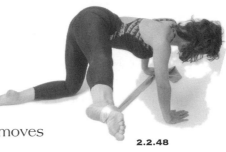

2.2.48

5. STRAIGHT LEG SIDE LIFT

a. From the all-fours position, stretch the R leg behind you and move it
to the side (toes still on the floor). (2.2.47)

b. Lift your leg as high in the air as is comfortable, then lower it again
to the floor. (2.2.49)

c. Repeat the leg lifts the number of times that is appropriate to you.

• The working leg remains straight as you lift and lower it to the
side.

d. Reach the leg behind you and return the leg to the all-fours position.

• Keep the weight on both arms equally.

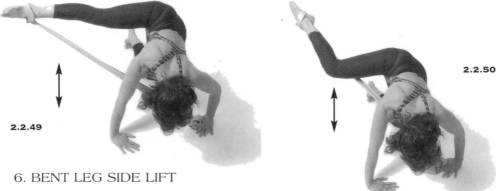

2.2.50

2.2.49

6. BENT LEG SIDE LIFT

a. From the all-fours position, lift
your R leg in the air to the side while it is bent at the knee. (2.2.50)

b. Lower it to the floor to the starting position.

• Be sure to stay evenly supported on both arms.

7. FULL HEAD/TAIL ARCH

a. Lengthen your R leg behind you by sliding it on the floor; then lift it
off the floor.

- Lift your leg as high as is comfortable for you.

b. Arch your back with your head and eyes facing upward to continue the arch. (2.2.51)

c. Return to all-fours position.

d. Bring your R leg back in and underneath your body, curving the back and drawing the R knee and head toward each other. (2.2.52)

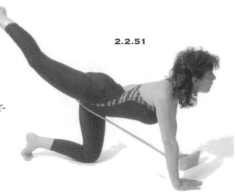

2.2.51

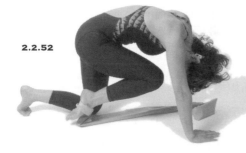

2.2.52

e. Repeat this exercise with the working leg in a turned-out position.

NOTE: On the return, as the leg comes under your chest, turn the leg back to parallel.

8. SECOND SIDE: Change the band to the L foot and repeat all parts on the second side.

NOTE: The following exercise may be done as an extension of #1–8, or entirely separate from them.

9. SOLE LIFT

STARTING POSITION: In the all-fours position on your hands and knees.

a. Raise the R leg behind you to the height of your back, keeping your leg in a parallel position.

b. Bend the R knee to create a 90° angle from your lower leg to thigh.

c. Flex your R foot, so the sole faces the ceiling. (2.2.53)

2.2.53

- Your abdominals should support your lower back by pulling in toward your spine and up toward your ribs.

BAND: One loop is attached to the R foot and the band runs along the outside of the leg and is held by the R hand. As an alternative it may also run beside the body and under it, held in the L hand. (2.2.53)

EXERCISE

    a. Slowly lift the sole of your R foot toward the ceiling, moving the leg in the hip socket. (2.2.53)

    b. Lower it until the thigh is even with the back.

- Keep the knee bent at 90°. Make sure the knee of your R leg stays abducted toward the midline of your body.
- In the starting position, your knee, hip, and shoulder should be aligned with each other.

    c. You may repeat the exercise with the band going over the body and held in the opposite hand.

    d. SECOND SIDE: Change the band to the L foot and repeat all parts on the second side.

NOTE: Rest your lower back by kneeling and folding your body in with your head on the floor and your hips on your heels.

VI. THE LITTLE MERMAID'S TAIL (Hip/Leg Rotation)

POSITION: Sit in fourth position (See Appendix C, #4 on page 170) with your L leg bent in front of your body and your R leg bent behind you. (2.2.54)

- This will create an open square between the inner sides of your R and L thighs.
- Your R knee should be behind you as much as is comfortable.

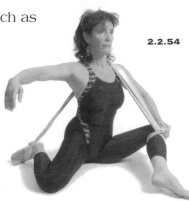

2.2.54

The same hand as your back leg will rest on the foot of your forward leg, and the other one will be either on the knee of your forward leg or beside it on the ground.

- Make sure your back is supported in the most erect position possible.

BAND: Attach one end of the band to your pointed R foot. Have the band come diagonally across the back and over the L shoulder. Wrap it once or twice around your lower leg, right below the L knee to stabilize the band.

- Begin each part of the exercise with your R leg rotated inward, so that the foot is lifted into the air while the thigh remains on the ground. (2.2.55)

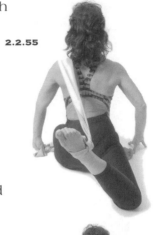

2.2.55

EXERCISE:

1. SIMPLE

   a. Lower your R lower leg and foot toward the floor, using your R knee as the pivot point. (2.2.56)

   b. Lift your R lower leg and foot upward to the starting position. (2.2.55)

     • Allow your pelvis to rotate slightly backward as your foot presses down to the floor so that both sitting bones are on the floor.

     • Rotate forward as your foot lifts up again.

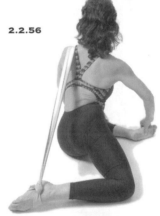

2.2.56

   c. Repeat parts a. and b., above, except the movement of the leg and hip will be isolated. That is, the movement will take place entirely in the hip joint. Do a smaller movement with the leg if you need to, as long as your hip remains fixated where it is as your L lower leg lifts up.

2. BACK LEG EXTENSION

   a. Straighten your R leg directly behind you. Extend it in an elongated line aligned behind the R side of your back. (2.2.57)

     • As your foot reaches out along the floor (in an arabesque), your knee will lift off the floor.

   b. Return the working leg to its starting position, using your bent R knee as a hinge to bend the lower leg back to the beginning position.

     • As you return from the extended line, allow your R knee to come softly to the floor.

   c. Repeat a. and b. several times.

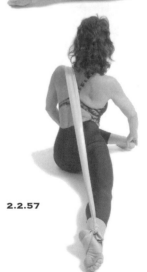

2.2.57

3. TRANSITION TO THE SECOND SIDE
   a. Extend your lower R leg behind you in a straight line. Let the knee drop gently down on the floor.
   b. Rotate your R hip out to let the R leg rotate and the R knee come up toward the ceiling, and use your hands behind you for support.
      • This will rotate your body halfway to the side.
   c. Let go of the band and, with both knees bent and together, curve your back and rest your lower back as long as needed.
   d. Change the band to the other foot.
   e. Rotate another quarter of a turn to the L side, and you will end up in the same position in which you started, only facing the opposite direction.
      • Your R leg is now in front. Now, you are ready to do the other side.

NOTE: In each stage of the exercise, try to bring your knee back a little farther behind you.

4. SECOND SIDE: Change the band to the L foot and repeat all parts on the second side.

VII. STRENGTHENING THE ADDUCTORS

POSITION: Sit in fourth position with your L leg forward and your R leg behind, as in VI: THE LITTLE MERMAID'S TAIL, on page 79. After you've attached the band, lean back so your weight is on both hands equally.

BAND: Attach one end to the pointed L foot. Then, stretch the other end over the R shoulder and hold it the L hand on the floor directly behind you. Be sure the band is taut enough to challenge you.

EXERCISE:

1. SIMPLE
   a. Lift your L leg (the front leg) in an wide angle, slightly bent at the knee.
      • Keep the leg turned out at the hip.
   b. Slowly, lower your R leg down toward the floor. (2.2.58)
      • Try to keep your ankle and knee on the same level, parallel to the floor.

81

- Scoop the abdominals for support. Do not allow your torso to sink down into the pelvis to achieve more height.

c. Repeat several times.

2. LIFT AND EXTENSION

a. Lift the front leg as in #1: SIMPLE on page 81.

b. Extend the leg forward (a ballet développé devant). (2.2.59)

- The working leg will straighten.

- Work very slowly and concentrate on keeping the heel up and leg turned out.

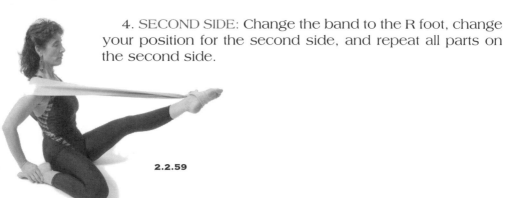

2.2.58

c. Bring the leg back to the bent angle with the same control (as in a.).

- Let your knee be a hinge so that the lower leg moves to reach the line of the thigh.

d. Repeat b. and c. several times.

e. Either return the L leg to the floor starting position, or continue with #3.

3. EXTENSION SIDE

a. Lift the front leg as in #1: SIMPLE.

b. Open the L knee farther to the side and extend the leg to the side.

- Turn your neck toward the leg so that the band does not cut you.

c. Bend your leg to return to the in-air, bent-leg shape.

d. Repeat a. and b.

4. SECOND SIDE: Change the band to the R foot, change your position for the second side, and repeat all parts on the second side.

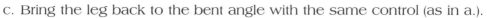

2.2.59

VIII. THE PENDULUM (Hip/Leg Rotation)

POSITION:

    a. Lie on your back. Legs are bent with knees facing up. Both feet are on the floor.

    b. With the R leg bent, raise it up to your chest.

    c. Allow your R leg to open up naturally on a diagonal to the R side while still keeping the knee bent at the same angle. (2.2.60)

        • Be sure the L side is stable and on the floor.

BAND: Attach one or both loops to your pointed R foot and hold the band in your L hand.

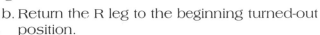

2.2.60

EXERCISE:

    a. Using your knee as a pivot point, lower the R lower leg and foot down to the floor underneath you by rotating the thigh inward from the hip joint. (2.2.61)

        • As your lower leg rotates down, your L knee does not change the height you set at the beginning.

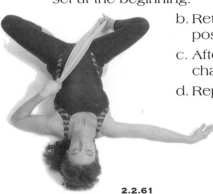

    b. Return the R leg to the beginning turned-out position.

    c. After several repetitions, lying on your back, change the band to the L foot.

    d. Repeat a. and b. on the second side.

2.2.61

IX. LEG ADDUCTORS

POSITION: Lie on your back. Bend your knees, drawing them up to your chest. Then, keeping your knees bent, open your legs wide naturally.

BAND: Attach one end of the band to each foot. Then cross the band and hold it with both hands at the center of the chest (sternum) at a point on the band that will provide you with the appropriate amount of resistance. Your elbows are on the floor for stabilization. (2.2.62)

EXERCISE:

a. Open the lower part of both legs to make a straight line from the hips to the toes, creating a "V" with your legs. Feet are flexed.

   • Leave the thighs and knees where they are.
   • The pelvis will lift slightly off the ground as you move.
   • Feet are flexed on the stretch open and pointed in the starting position. As an alternative, the feet may be pointed the whole time. (2.2.63)

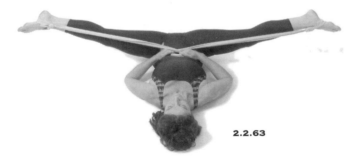

2.2.62

2.2.63

b. Return to the starting position with pointed feet.
c. Repeat as needed for your exercise program.
d. Repeat steps a. and b. above, with the pelvis remaining on the ground.
e. Close the bent legs, pull them to your chest, and rest.

X. ANTIGRAVITY FOOT WORK

POSITION:

1. Lie on your back with your legs straight up in the air at a 90° angle. Feet are flexed. (2.2.64)

   • You may use a wall, if needed.

   • Your legs should not lean forward toward the face.

2. Turn your legs out at the hip joint, so the feet are in a turned-out first position—the heels are together. (2.2.65)

3. Point the feet.

4. Bend your knees into a diamond shape. (2.2.66)

2.2.64

BAND: Place one end of the band on each foot. Cross the band in front of the shins and hold it at center of your torso. The elbows are bent and wide apart, pulling the band toward the floor.

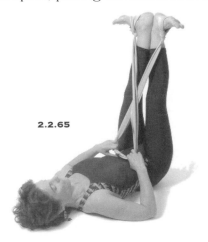

2.2.65

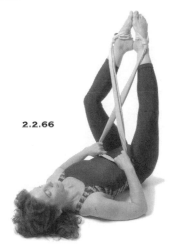

2.2.66

EXERCISE:

1. SIMPLE

   a. Keep your knees bent (plié) while you flex both feet.

   b. Point both feet.

   c. Repeat for as many repetitions as you need.

2. POINT-FLEX ALTERNATING

   a. With straight legs (at a 90° angle), alternate the action of the feet:

as the R leg bends and the R foot flexes, the L leg and foot remain extended and pointed. (2.2.67)

3. FOOT CIRCLES

NOTE: Move away from the wall if you have been using one.

OUTWARD CIRCLES

    a. With legs straight, circle one foot at a time in a slow, full, outward circle—first the R foot, then the L foot.

    b. Circle both feet outward at the same time. (not on video)

INWARD CIRCLES

    a. As in steps a. and b. directly above (Outward Circles), except the circles will be inward instead of outward.

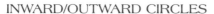

2.2.67

INWARD/OUTWARD CIRCLES

    a. Circle your R foot inward while you circle your L foot outward.

    b. Repeat, changing the directions of the feet.

NOTE: The difference between the video and the book represents slightly different versions of the same exercise. Both are correct.

XI. CALF AND FOOT: REVVING THE ACCELERATOR (Working against a Chair)

POSITION: Lie on your back in front of a wall with your R knee bent at a 90° angle (as if you were resting it on a chair seat), with the sole of your R foot flat against the wall. (2.2.68)

NOTE: If you do not have wall space, you can use a chair that is the right height for you, with your R leg resting on the seat of a chair and the sole of your R foot against the chair back (not pictured). Anchor the chair against a wall to keep it steady as you work.

BAND: Place both ends of the band in the middle part (metatarsals) of R foot. Run the band along both sides of the R calf.

1. BEGINNER: Hold one strand of the band in the R hand at the R side

2.2.68

of your calf; hold the other strand of the band in the L hand at the
L side of your calf. (2.2.68)

2. ADVANCED: Run both strands of the band along
the inside of your R leg. Use your L hand to hold the
center of the band. With your R arm extended toward
your hips on the floor or out to the side, your
R hand will help to stabilize your body.

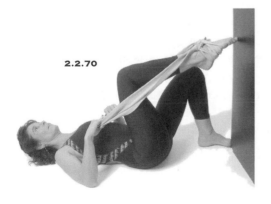

EXERCISE:

1. SIMPLE

    a. Raise your heel away from the
       wall or chair back (ballet relevé). (2.2.69)

       • Make sure all five toes are still attached to the wall or chair back.

    b. Return slowly to having the full sole of the foot on the wall or chair.

    c. Repeat a. and b. several times.

2. FULL FOOT EXTENSION

    a. Raise your heel away from the wall or chair back and extend the
       toes to full-pointe, so that your big toe is hardly touching the chair
       back or wall. (2.2.70)

    b. Slowly, go through the position where your toes are resting on the
       chair back or wall. Flatten the sole of the foot on the chair back again.

    c. Place your R foot higher on the chair or wall and repeat a. and b.

    d. Fixate the heel against the chair and allow the toes and the center
       of the foot to flex. (2.2.71)

    e. Return to starting position.

3. SECOND SIDE: Change the band to the L foot, change the leg positions,
and repeat all parts on the second side.

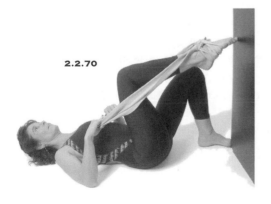

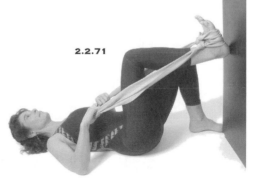

XII. THE STORK LEG WORK

POSITION: Stand with your feet parallel and about hips-width apart. Bend your knees slightly. Bent elbows are outward with hands on hips.

BAND: Place one end of the band on the L foot. Spread the center of the band over your L shoulder and hold the other end with your R hand on your R hip.

NOTE:

a. Throughout this exercise, the supporting leg is extremely important. You need to "climb" out of it. Do not sink into it.

b. Make sure your supporting leg's knee is not hyperextended (locked).

c. Be sure to keep the tailbone directed down to the floor. Do not tuck.

d. The bottom of the pelvis (sitting bones or iscial tuberosities) remain even throughout.

EXERCISE:

1. TENDU AND DÉVELOPPÉ FRONT:

a. Lift the flexed L foot to knee height (passé), next to the R knee. (2.2.72)

b. Extend your L leg approximately 15° diagonally forward. (2.2.73)

• Keep your foot flexed; your heel should touch the floor.

• Allow your hip to rise on a. and sink on b. as you do the movement.

c. Return to the flexed L foot to knee height (passé).

d. Repeat b. and c., above, fixating the pelvis.

• The leg will work separately from the hip. That is, do not allow your hip to rise and sink as you do the movement.

e. With a flexed foot, develop your L leg to an extension to thigh height—90° or as high as you can—in the air in front of you. (2.2.74)

• Leg remains parallel.

• Allow the pelvis to rise and fall with the movement.

• The height of your leg will depend upon your flexibility, and how high you lifted the thigh.

2.2.72

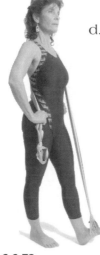

2.2.73

f. Return to the flexed L foot to knee height (passé).

g. Extend the L leg front with the foot extended (pointed).

h. Return to the flexed-foot passé.

i. Lower the L leg to stand on it.

2. TENDU AND DÉVELOPPÉ SIDE

a. Lift the flexed L foot to knee height (passé).

b. Extend the bent leg 15° diagonally to the side. (2.2.75)

• Leg is parallel and to the side, foot flexed.

• Most people are not able to open their leg exactly to the side of the body, so you may open your leg on a diagonal between front and side if necessary.

2.2.74

c. Return to the flexed L foot to knee height (passé).

d. Extend the L leg side to 15° with the foot extended (pointed).

e. Return to the flexed L foot to knee height (passé).

f. Repeat b.–d. with a fixed pelvis (moving the leg independent of the pelvis).

g. Repeat b.–e. with a higher leg and fixed pelvis.

h. Lower the L leg to stand on it.

2.2.75

3. TENDU AND DÉVELOPPÉ BACK

a. Lift the flexed L foot to knee height (passé).

b. Extend the bent leg behind you to approximately 15° (tendu). Your heel leads. (2.2.76)

c. Return to the flexed L foot to knee height (passé).

d. Extend the L leg back with the foot extended (pointed).

e. Return to the flexed L foot to knee height (passé).

f. Repeat b.–e. with a fixed pelvis (moving the leg independent of the pelvis).

g. Lift the leg to full height behind you, flexed foot.

h. Return to the flexed L foot to knee height (passé).

i. Lift the leg to full height behind you, pointed foot.

j. Return to the flexed L foot to knee height (passé).

k. Lower the L leg to stand on it.

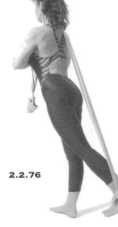

2.2.76

4. TURNED OUT

BAND: The band runs on the outside of the working leg.

   a. Repeat the five exercises above with the thigh of the working leg turned out instead of parallel. (2.2.77, 2.2.78, and 2.2.79)

   • Supporting leg can stay parallel.

   • Turning out the supporting leg makes the exercise more advanced.

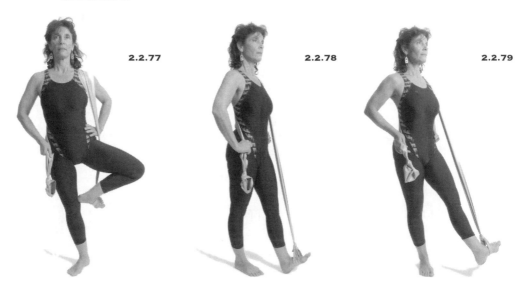

2.2.77   2.2.78   2.2.79

5. WITH POINTED FOOT

   a. Repeat all the above exercises (with the working leg in turned-in and turned-out positions) with the foot of the working leg pointed instead of flexed.

   • Throughout the exercises, the supporting leg is extremely important, and you need to "climb" out of it. That is, "pull out" of the pelvis instead of sinking into the bones and muscles.

   • Make sure your knee is not hyperextended (locked backward).

   • The tailbone should be directed down to the floor. Do not "tuck."

   • The sitting bones must stay at the same height from the floor and must be on the same level as well.

6. SECOND SIDE: Change the band to the R foot and repeat all parts on the second side.

7. VARIATIONS: You may do all of these exercises with the first leg working only with a flexed foot and then with a pointed foot.

Lessons from Life

#1. NOWHERE

To be where there is no movement and no touch is a horrifying thought.

#2. MOVEMENT IS EVERYWHERE

Movement is everywhere. It is always happening, whether we think about it or not. Try this: Stand still for a minute and pay attention. There is so much that goes on. Were you even aware of it? For example, can you sense the tendons running along each side of your ankle? There are many indiscernible readjustments that happen every moment in order to support your body and stabilize your balance.

#3. BALANCE

Balance is a very significant word for me. This is illustrated in my five-year-old daughter's first visit to the dentist. Remembering my experiences, I knew a child's first trip to the dentist requires psychological preparation. The dentist was kind. At the outset, he allowed her to handle some of his instruments, the small mirrors, the air jet and water syringe. As part of his philosophy, he also allowed her to establish the tempo for all that would happen to her. While appreciating her enjoyment, the dentist said, "What a bright-eyed little girl you have." I replied, "Is that unusual?" "Oh yes," he said, "so many of them have eyes of blah." "Blah," I asked? "Eyes like glass," he continued. "Comes from hours and hours of watching TV." As you can see *balance* is a very important word for me.

#4. SCAFFOLDING

When teaching about the torso muscles initiating movements, or the idea of crossing the band—with the band from the right foot held in the left hand and vice versa, I imagine the shape of a building's scaffold, with the beams crossed in an "x" shape to give it support and strength.

#5. FINDING NUTRITIONAL BALANCE

We are bombarded with nutritional information from nutritionists, books, and television telling us we must have a balanced diet. We must have the proper amount of protein, starch, fat, milk, fruits, and vegetables, each day. Each authority sets forth his or her own set of measures. This confused me. In addition, I was forever getting hung up on "Yes, but . . ." A case in point: a banana is a fruit, but it is also starch, so where do I categorize it? In the end, I had to find my own *balance*. To me, *balance* has come to mean "stay simple." Separate foods. For example, after a lunch made of peanut butter (protein) on whole grain bread (starch) I feel tired. On the other hand, protein by itself in one meal and starch, in the next, is easier on my digestive system. For me, separation is proper balance. Each person must find his or her own balance.

#6. HANDWRITING AND BODY HABITS

Each one of us has a different hand signature and a specific, unique handwriting. What exactly makes this so? Some psychology experts say that there are personality traits that explain this phenomenon, but physiologically, we each differ in how we hold our pen and how we move our fingers to create the letter shape. The amount of pressure that our pen needs to put ink on the paper also varies.

#7. FELT MOVEMENT

Have you ever stepped off a moving train or ship onto solid ground? Remember how the movement of the ship and feeling of inner rocking stayed with you for hours? I enjoy that unusual inner space.

#8. TEACHER PAYBACK

As a teacher, I find it is often difficult to know how much of what I teach is actually being absorbed by my students. One year, at the end of the semester, I asked my students in the Dance Department at the University of South Florida to come up with one thing they learned about themselves from taking my class.

I remember a particular dancer who brought some of her own shoes for this assignment, as a kind of "show-and-tell" demonstration. First, she showed the class a pair of flat-heeled shoes that had a clear imprint of her foot on the front part of the inner soles. She made the connection between her posture and the way her weight was distributed on her feet. She also showed a pair of yellow shoes with very high heels. She used these shoes to explain how the height of the heel could account for the tightness and shortness of her hamstring muscles. I went home smiling that day.

#9. ARCHES

Have your ever seen the beautiful arches in the ceilings of the ancient European churches or the arches of the Roman aqueduct? Your bones have the same arched inner structure. Taking that thought farther, stand up. Put your feet together, side by side. Look at them. Can you see the arches of your feet creating a dome shape? Can you see the strength and support that is carried up your legs and into your pelvic floor? Can you see the benefit of this support?

#10. SLINKY AND YOU

Do you remember playing with the toy made from a coiled wire spring—a Slinky? Think of how fluently it moved when you pushed it gently from the top of the stairs and it began to ripple down the steps, turning end over end, until it reached the bottom. Remember how it looked when you held it from the top ring and let it spiral down toward the floor. We can apply the spiral principle of the Slinky to standing up with more efficient use of energy. The next time you get up from a chair, try to imitate that same spiral pattern. Place one foot slightly in front of the other, then think of rotating your hips and shifting your weight over your feet as you rise. Do you feel the ease of doing this as opposed to trying to just "power" your way to a standing position? Try the same thing from sitting on the floor in a crossed-legged position, basically leaving the feet in the same place where they are at the start. For example, if your right foot is in front as you sit, you will cross the right foot over the left knee. Begin to rotate the hip and torso to the left while pushing with the left hand into the floor behind you. Turn the head and eyes upward to the left to precede the body. Keep a low center of gravity to hold your balance. By the time you have rotated into a standing position, you will have made a complete half-turn to face the opposite direction.

#11. BODY RE-EDUCATION

The nervous system is like a governor. In other words, it should receive the attention and intention we put into the body. If we find a way to re-educate our bodies to perform better-quality movement, we can uncover unfinished stages in our developmental progress. For example, relearn how to crawl with opposition between the right leg and the left arm. Doing this will correct our difficulties originating at that time of development. Your nervous system, in conjunction with your brain, has the extraordinary power to improve, heal, and allow choices of movement in the body.

#12. WALK/IDENTIFY

I remember one Tuesday afternoon that I had off from army camp. I rushed to the city to pamper myself, so I could feel a little feminine again. By the time it was dark, I saw an unclear image of a person moving, walking a couple of blocks in front of me. I looked again, and it suddenly hit me. I thought to myself, "Oh yeah, that's my mom!" I went forward to greet her. I had not seen her for a month. From that distance, in the dim light, it would seem to be impossible to tell for sure who it was. So how did I know? The first thing I recognized was her walk. I saw her familiar head swing, and the movement of her shoulders up and down, forward and back. You may have had the same experience as well, knowing who someone was simply because of the way they walk. Perhaps you did not break it down into its elements at the time, but somehow, you just knew. When we walk, we all make unconscious choices of how to use our body. What is your shoulder movement (or lack of movement) when you lift the opposite hip? As you take a step do you move your pelvis, or do you swing from your legs down? Do your shoulders move up and down, forward and back with each step? How much do your knees bend?

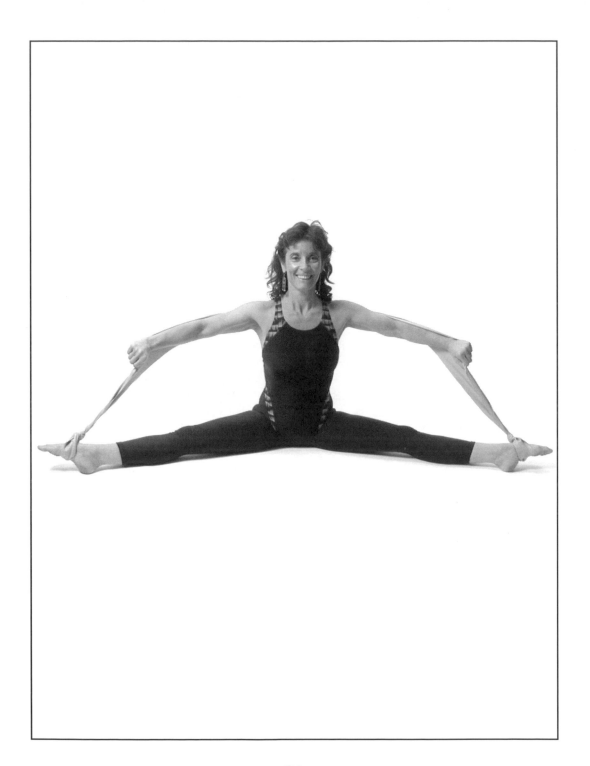

Chapter 2

Chapter Two: Exercises

PART 3: UPPER BODY

Human beings are
soft and supple when alive,
stiff and straight when dead.

The myriad creatures, the grasses and trees are
soft and fragile when alive,
dry and withered when dead.

Therefore it is said:
The rigid person is a disciple of death; the soft, supple, and delicate are lovers of life.

An army that is inflexible will not conquer; A tree that is inflexible will snap.

The unyielding and mighty shall be brought low;
The soft, supple, and delicate will be set above.

> — Lao Tzu
> *Tao Te Ching* (1990: 52)

MUSCLES OF THE SHOULDER JOINT

1. Deltoids (2.3.1)

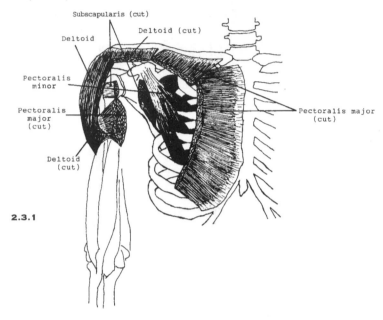

2.3.1

2. Supraspinatus (2.3.2)

3. Infraspinatus (2.3.2 and 2.3.4)

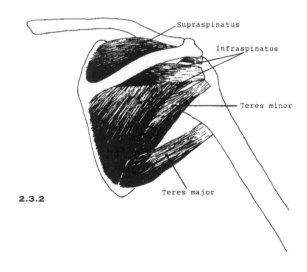

2.3.2

4. Subscapularis (2.3.1)

5. Teres major (2.3.2 and 2.3.4)

6. Latissimus dorsi (2.3.4 and 2.3.6)

7. Pectoralis major (2.3.1)

MUSCLES OF THE ARM

1. Biceps brachii (2.3.3.)

2. Brachialis (2.3.3.)

3. Brachioradialis (2.3.3.)

4. Triceps (2.3.3.)

5. Pronator teres (2.3.3.)

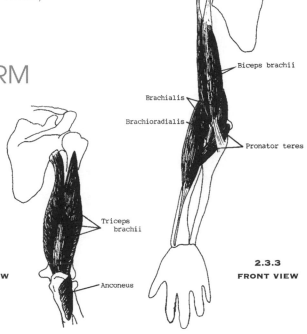

Biceps brachii

Brachialis

Brachioradialis

Pronator teres

2.3.3
FRONT VIEW

Triceps
brachii

Anconeus

2.3.3
BACK VIEW

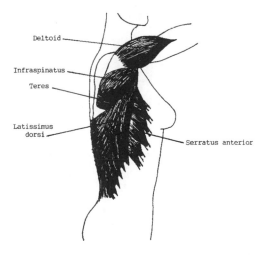

Deltoid

Infraspinatus

Teres

Latissimus
dorsi

Serratus anterior

2.3.4

97

MUSCLES OF THE LATERAL TORSO

1. Serratus anterior (2.3.4)
2. Quadratus lumborum (2.1.4 - pg. 41)
3. Obliquus externus abdominis (2.1.2 - pg. 40)
4. Obliquus internus abdominis (2.1.3 - pg. 40)
5. Internal intercostal
6. External intercostal

MUSCLES OF THE SHOULDER GIRDLE

1. Trapezius (2.3.5)
2. Levator scapula (2.3.6)
3. Rhomboids (2.3.6)
4. Serratus anterior (2.3.4)
5. Pectoralis minor (2.3.4)

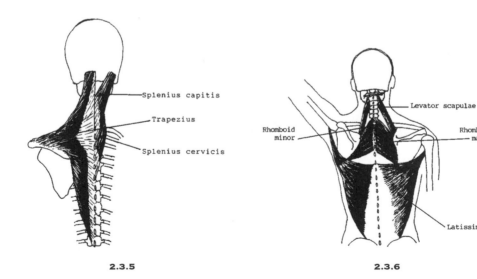

2.3.5

2.3.6

I. CHEST PRESS

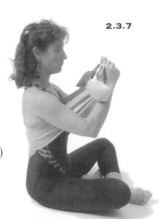

2.3.7

POSITION: Stand, sit, or kneel with the upper arms at the sides of the body. Bend the elbows to a 90° angle forward, with the upper arms parallel to the floor and to each other.

BAND: Run the band across the shoulder blades (scapulae) and under the armpits. Hold the band in each hand at a place on the band that will provide you with the appropriate amount of resistance. (2.3.7)

EXERCISE:

1. SIMPLE

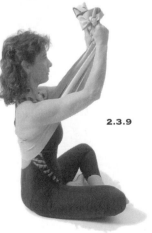

2.3.8

  a. With the palms facing the floor or facing each other, press the arms and hands directly forward so that the arms are extended in front of you. (2.3.8)

   b. Return to the starting position. (2.3.7)

   c. Repeat, trying to press the arms forward an inch higher each time. (2.3.9)

   d. Once you work up to the highest diagonal, hold your arms out in the extended position.

   e. Lower and raise your arms in front of you so that your shoulder joint acts as a hinge.

   • Be sure to keep the shoulder blades depressed. (2.3.10)

   f. Repeat several times.

2. BENT ARM RAISE

  a. Keeping the elbows in the same 90° angle and pushing the elbows away from the body, raise the arms so the upper arm is next to your head.

   • At completion, the upper arms should be perpendicular to the floor and the

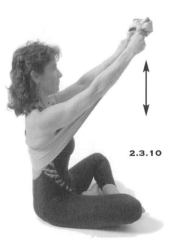

2.3.9

2.3.10

lower arms should be parallel to the floor and behind your back.

- Keep the ribs in throughout.

b. Return to the starting position.

c. Repeat several times.

II. THE SHAWL

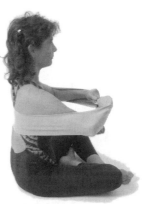

POSITION

a. Sit comfortably, crossed legs in front of you.

b. Bend your arms at the elbows and hold your hands a small distance in front of your chest.

c. Lift the elbows to each side and turn your hands slightly outward, so the backs of your hands are facing toward you. (2.3.11)

BAND: For the "Shawl position," place the center of the band on your spine. The rest of the band wraps behind each elbow. Hold the band with each hand at a point that is comfortable for you.

2.3.11

- Try to position the elbows right in the middle of the band so the band does not slide.

- It takes a bit of practice to be able to place and hold the band behind the elbow.

EXERCISE:

1. SIMPLE, EXTENSION SIDE

a. Using the elbow as a hinge and keeping both elbows lifted, open and extend the hands and forearms out to the side. (2.3.12)

b. Return slowly.

c. Repeat a. and b., above, with the palms and fingers turned in to face you. (not on video)

2.3.12

2. SIMPLE: EXTENSION FORWARD

STARTING POSITION: Same starting position as SIMPLE, EXTENSION SIDE.

a. With the palms facing outward, extend the arms directly forward without locking the elbows. (2.3.13)

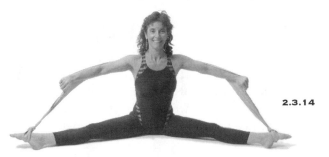

- The body will feel as though the torso is going back as the arms go forward.

b. Return slowly.

c. Repeat a. and b. above, with the palms and fingers turned in to face you. (not on video)

3. SHAWL VARIATION (not on video)

STARTING POSITION: Sit in a wide parallel second position on the floor with your feet pointed.

- Your knees will face the ceiling.

2.3.13

BAND: Attach each end of the band to each foot with the center of the band behind your back, passing underneath the scapula. Stretch the band above the elbows, which are bent slightly toward the back. Hold the band with each hand to stabilize it. (2.3.14)

2.3.14

EXERCISE:

1. Contract your abdominals, letting your head and spine curve over (as if you were looking at your belly button) and allow the top of your pelvis to roll backward.
   - Make sure you lift your elbows and widen your back. (2.3.15)

2. Lengthen your arms out toward your feet.

3. Return to the starting position by lifting the pelvis back to its erect position, rolling the spine up, and bending the elbows.

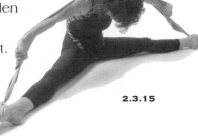

2.3.15

III. CRESCENT BEND

POSITION:

1. Straighten both your arms overhead at a distance that is a little wider than shoulder width. (2.3.16)

2. Legs are parallel, about hips-width apart.

NOTE: You will be lying in this position on the floor in the first exercise. All other exercises will be done in a standing position.

BAND: Hold the band near the ends but before the loops, one in each hand, with the band stretched. When you stand, the ends of the band will hang down on each side of your arms.

EXERCISE:

1. SIMPLE: ON THE FLOOR

STARTING POSITION: Lie on the floor in the position described above.

a. Keeping the R arm stationary (where it starts on the floor), pull your L arm down to the L side as the body curves into a crescent shape. (2.3.17)

 • Think of bending vertebra by vertebra, all the way down to the pelvis, without actually shifting the pelvis from center.

b. Slowly return to the starting position by bringing the L arm to the R arm (overhead), and leading with the R ribs.

 • Allow your chin to follow the head as the L arm extends the band.

 • It is okay if parts of the back do not touch the floor. Try to keep it as low to the floor as possible.

 • You may bend your knees if they feel overly stressed.

 • Do not release your abdominal muscles or rib cage.

c. Repeat on the second side.

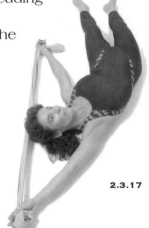

2.3.17

2. SIMPLE, STANDING—RIBS LEAD

STARTING POSITION: Stand in parallel first position in the position described above.

a. Repeat #1: SIMPLE, above, while standing in parallel first position.

- The band will stretch behind your head. (2.3.18)
- You will initiate the moving up to the starting position with your R ribs.

3. SIMPLE, STANDING: ARM LEADS RETURN

a. Begin as in #2: SIMPLE, STANDING, above, bending to the side.

b. Having bent your torso over to the L side, reach the R arm up toward the ceiling. (2.3.19)

- This is instead of initiating the rolling up from the R ribs.
- This creates the feeling of the R arm pulling you up to the starting position.

c. Repeat on the second side.

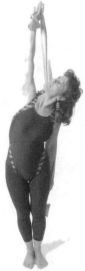

2.3.18

2.3.19

4. SIMPLE, STANDING: TORSO LEADS RETURN

a. In the standing position, bend to the side with your arms maintaining their same distance to each other and to your head.

- R arm also reaches L.

b. For an extra stretch, bend and straighten your knees.

c. Instead of initiating the rolling up from the ribs or the arm, think of lifting the whole torso up as a single unit.

- Do not allow your torso to tilt forward as you bend to the side. Keep your body facing directly to the front.
- Lengthen the arms outward, press down the scapulae, and maintain your torso in that position.
- Keep your rib cage in.

d. Repeat a.–c. on the second side.

103

5. VARIATIONS (not on video)

    a. Have your head face down or up to work different muscle groups in your neck and shoulders during the exercises. (2.3.20)

    b. Bend your knees to increase the difficulty during the exercises.

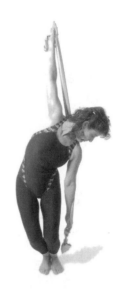

2.3.20

IV. HANDS OF THE CLOCK

POSITION: Sit or kneel in any comfortable position on the floor or on the edge of a chair, making certain that both sides of your body remain equal.

BAND: Hold the band above your head slightly wider than shoulder width apart and a little behind the head, so the arms act as an extension of the back. Keep your shoulder blades depressed as much as possible. (2.3.21)

• Be sure to keep the hand and forearm in alignment.

• Keep the scapulae down (not up toward your ears) in all positions.

2.3.21

EXERCISE:

NOTE: For each exercise, your L arm will remain in a constant position.

    1. HEAD ALONE

       a. Stretch your head and neck up, extending them.

       b. Then create an arch by moving your head toward your R arm, leading with the R ear. (2.3.22)

- Your nose will face *forward* during the entire exercise.
- Your arms do not move.

c. Return to upright.

d. Repeat a.–c. on the second side.

2. ARMS ALONE

a. Depress the R shoulder blade, and lift your R arm up toward your ear. (2.3.23)

b. Return your arm to the starting position.

c. Repeat a. and b. on the second side.

2.3.22

3. COMBINATION OF SIMPLE, #1 and 2

a. The head will arch down to the R side. The R arm will lift, and both will meet at the center of the arch.

- Depress the shoulder blades each time you raise or lower your arms.
- Keep the eyes and nose focused forward.
- Do not protrude the ribs forward.

b. Return the head to upright and the arm to the V-shape overhead.

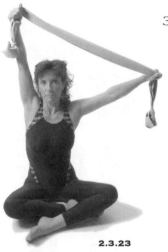

2.3.23

V. BICEPS

POSITION: Stand with the L foot slightly ahead of the R. Brace the R upper arm against the body and bend the lower arm to a 90° angle.

- For more stretch, start with the whole arm down at your side (as on the video).

BAND: Wrap one loop of the band around the L foot. Hold the other end in the L hand with the palm facing up.

EXERCISE:

a. Keeping the L elbow held against the body, bring the L palm, wrist, and forearm up, toward the L shoulder. (2.3.24)

b. Slowly return to starting position.

• Do not bend your wrist while doing the exercise.

• Keep the working palm facing up.

c. Repeat several times.

d. Change the band and stance for the second side and repeat the exercise.

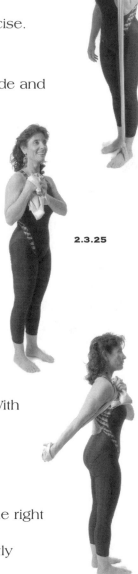

2.3.24

2.3.25

2.3.26

VI. TRICEPS

POSITION:

a. Stand with legs and feet parallel to each other.

b. Bend the R arm close to your side, so that your R hand is near the R shoulder and the arm is braced at the ribs.

c. Bend the L arm, and hold it at the R shoulder or in front of your chest. (2.3.25)

d. Hold the R hand against the R shoulder.

BAND: Hold both ends of the band in your L hand, which will remain stationary throughout the exercise. With your R hand, hold the doubled band at a point that will provide you with the appropriate amount of resistance.

EXERCISE:

1. ARM EXTENSION DOWNWARD

a. Extend the right hand and arm down toward the right side of the body.

b. Continue this extension until the R arm is slightly behind the body. (2.3.26)

• You will be using the R elbow as a hinge.

c. Return slowly to starting position.

d. Repeat several times.

e. Change the band and repeat on the second side.

2. ARM EXTENSION UPWARD

STARTING POSITION: Place both hands either behind your head (2.3.27) or right above the pelvis. Continue to hold the band as in the BAND directions for this exercise.

NOTE: If this is too strong, you may hold the loop of the band in your L hand and the center of the band in your R hand.

a. Lengthen the L hand and forearm above the head. (2.3.28)

b. Return slowly to starting position.

c. Repeat several times.

d. Change the band and repeat a.–c. on the second side.

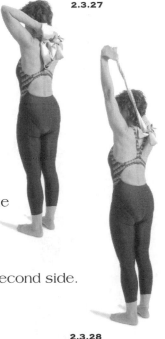

2.3.27

2.3.28

VII. THE TRAFFIC DIRECTOR

NOTE:

• Most of the exercises in this section can be done in either a sitting or in a standing position unless otherwise specified.

• You may do them in sections, or all at once.

POSITION: Hold the arms overhead a little wider than shoulder-width apart. Slightly bend the elbows. Palms forward.

• Rotate elbows backward to keep them from locking.

BAND: Hold the band with both hands over the head. (2.3.29)

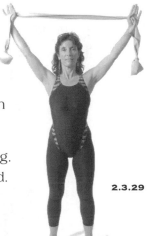

2.3.29

EXERCISE:

NOTE: To achieve the maximum results for the arm and back muscles, do each exercise once with the arm rotated in (palm and fingers facing down) and once with the arm rotated out (palm and fingers facing up when arms are directly in front of you).

1. OVERHEAD TO SHOULDER HEIGHT
   a. Exhale while slowly stretching the band directly to each side until the hands are at shoulder height.
      • The band will be stretched to your shoulders, just below your head. (2.3.30)

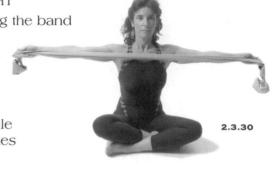

2.3.30

   b. Return arms to overhead while depressing the shoulder blades at the same time.
   c. Change the hands so that they face back and repeat a. and b.
   d. Repeat a.–c. above, stretching the band behind your body as you pull your arms to the sides. (2.3.31)

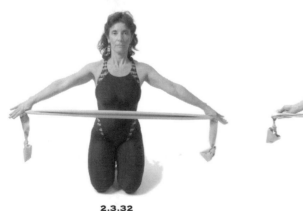

2.3.31

2. FRONT LOW TO SHOULDER HEIGHT

STARTING POSITION: Hold the band down in front of your body, to start. Palms face backward. (2.3.32)

   a. Extend both arms directly to each side, moving them upward until they are at shoulder height.
   b. Return arms to low.
   c. Change the band so that your palms face forward and repeat a. and b. (2.3.33)

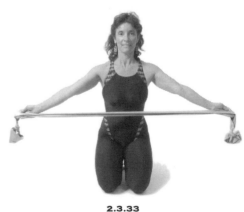

2.3.32   2.3.33

3. BACK LOW TO SHOULDER HEIGHT

STARTING POSITION: Hold the band low, behind your back, palms forward. (2.3.34)

a. Repeat #2: FRONT LOW TO SHOULDER HEIGHT, above, holding the band behind the body as you raise your arms.

b. Return arms to low back.

- Elbows turn and bend slightly.

- If you are standing, be sure your legs are slightly bent.

c. Repeat with palms turned to the back. (2.3.35)

NOTE: To vary the muscles being used, you can perform this exercise with one palm facing forward and one palm facing back.

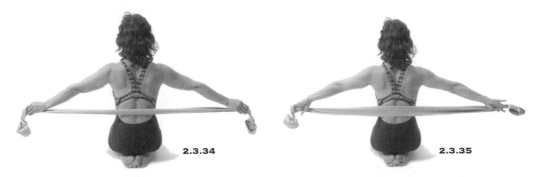

2.3.34   2.3.35

4. EXTEND SIDE, FROM FRONT

STARTING POSITION: Hold the band in both hands, palms down, and extend your arms directly forward. (2.3.36)

a. Open your arms to each side, keeping the same relationship between the arms and the body. (2.3.37)

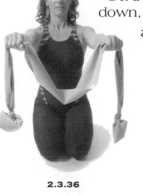

2.3.36

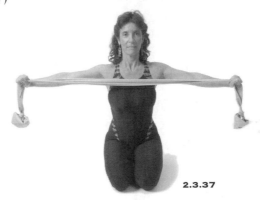

2.3.37

NOTE: Do not let the shoulder blades "pinch" together; instead, try to widen the back by thinking of your shoulder blades staying as far away from your spine as possible.

    b. Return to arms shoulder-width apart.

    c. Repeat a. and b. with palms up.

5. DIAGONALS

STARTING POSITION: In order to work the biceps, do the following three exercises holding the band with your palms up. Hold your palms down, if you wish to work the triceps. (2.3.38) Begin each variation with both arms extended directly forward, as in the #4: EXTEND SIDE, FROM FRONT, above.

2.3.38

BOTH ARMS MOVE

    a. Open the R arm to an upward diagonal and the L arm to a downward diagonal, both arms working at the same time.

    b. Return to the starting position.

      • Pay extra attention to controlling the shoulder blade (scapula) movement.

    c. Do the second side by reaching the L arm diagonally upward and the R arm diagonally downward.

    d. Change the directions of the palms and repeat a.–c.

ONE ARM MOVES

    a. Keep the L arm in the original position, directly forward. Isolate the R arm by lifting it up into a diagonal. (2.3.39)

      • This exercise will specifically work the triceps.

    b. Return to the starting position.

    c. Change the palm direction and reach up with the R arm again and return to the starting position

    d. Change the palm direction and reach down with the R arm. (2.3.40)

    e. Return to the starting position.

    f. Change the palm direction and reach down with the R arm and return.

    g. Repeat a.–f. with the R arm fixed and the L arm reaching up or reaching down.

2.3.39

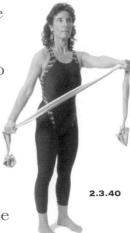

2.3.40

6. ROTATION (not on video)

NOTE: ROTATION may be last in your program. It puts all planes of movement together, and is good to use after flexion, extension, and abduction.

STARTING POSITION: Stand with the legs parallel, about hip-width apart. Raise the arms and hold the band above the head at about shoulder-width apart. (2.3.41)

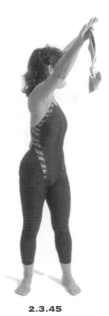

2.3.41

SIMPLE (not on video)

a. Rotate the upper body from the waist to face the L side; the hips remain facing forward. (2.3.42)

b. While moving into this position, stretch the band with both arms moving directly to each side, to about the height of your shoulders. (2.3.43)

c. Continue bringing the arms down in front of the L thigh. (2.3.44)

d. Rotate the upper body from the waist to the R side, hips still facing forward while reversing the arm movement. (2.3.45)

• You will end facing R with your arms overhead.

• Remember to keep the hips facing forward.

e. Rotate the torso to face directly forward, as in the beginning of this exercise.

NOTE: These photographs mirror your movement.

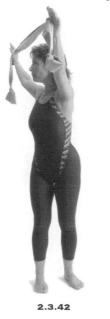
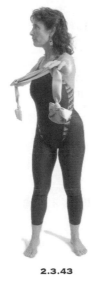
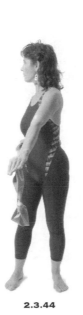
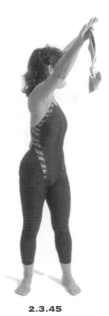

| 2.3.42 | 2.3.43 | 2.3.44 | 2.3.45 |

ADVANCED

a. Begin by twisting the body to the L. (2.3.42)

b. Roll your body down as you open your arms and lower them to shoulder height.

- Arms are to the side in relation to the body.

- Remember to keep the hips facing forward.

c. Continue moving the arms all the way down toward the thigh.

d. Rotate (untwist) your body forward as you reverse your arms and open them to the side again.

- You will end bending to the L with your whole body facing forward.

e. Come up to straight, lifting your arms overhead to the starting position.

f. Repeat a.–e. on the second side.

7. ABDUCTION (in the frontal plane)

STARTING POSITION: Place one end of the band on the R foot. Step forward slightly with the R foot, holding the band in the R hand down near your side at a point on the band that is comfortable for you.

ALTERNATIVE STARTING POSITIONS: If the starting position is too difficult for you, you may modify it these ways:

- From the R foot, stretch the band up behind you, over the R elbow, and over the R shoulder. The R hand holds the end of the band in front of the chest. You can now push the band out to the side with your elbow instead of the whole arm. You will find this to be easier since the lever (your arm) is half the length of the extended arm.

- (on the video) From the R foot, run the band from the back, up over your shoulder, and down to your R hand. The L hand holds the band to stabilize it at the R shoulder.

EXERCISE:

a. Lengthen the band upward, directly to the R side, as far as shoulder height.

b. Control the band as you return to the Starting Position.

2.3.46

c. Repeat several times.

d. Change the band and repeat on the second side.

- Be sure to exhale with the effort.

NOTE: A more difficult version is to simply hold the band in your R hand and stretch the arm and band to shoulder-height side. (2.3.46)

8. FLEXION

a. Repeat #7: ABDUCTION, above, except raise the R arm directly in front of you to shoulder height, instead of to the side. (2.3.47)

• This contracts your pectoralis muscle.

9. HORIZONTAL ABDUCTION/ADDUCTION

a. From the same starting position as #7: ABDUCTION, above, lift your arm to the side.

b. Next, move your arm from the side of the body to directly forward, then back to the side again. (2.3.48)

• Keep the same distance between the arm and body as you move (i.e., keep the arm extended and reaching outward).

• Be sure to exhale with the effort.

c. Repeat moving the whole arm from side to front to side several times.

d. Lower the arm.

e. Change the band and repeat a.–d. on the second side.

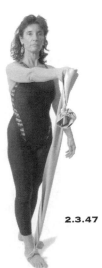

2.3.47

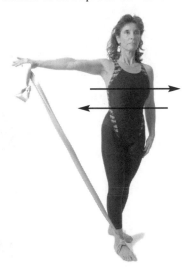

2.3.48

VIII. HEAD AND NECK: THE GIRAFFE

POSITION: Sit comfortably on your knees, cross-legged, or on a chair, as long as your body remains in good alignment.

BAND: You will be using the band against the head to create resistance for stretching and strengthening the neck and head muscles. Please note the position of the head for each individual exercise.

EXERCISE:

1. SIMPLE NECK STRETCH

BACK

BAND: Spread the width of the band behind your head and over your ears, and hold an end in each hand. (2.3.49)

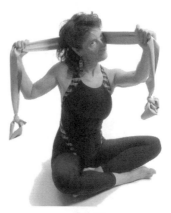

2.3.49

    a. Pull the band forward in front of your face as you push your nose and chin backward.

      • This will create a lengthening effect at the back of your neck.

    b. Repeat several times.

FRONT

BAND: Spread the width of the band across the forehead. (2.3.50)

    a. Pull the back backward slightly to create tension while you push your entire head forward.

      • Be sure not to pull just the chin.

    b. Repeat several times.

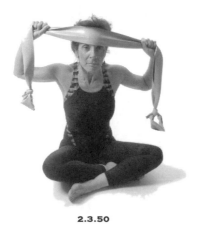

2.3.50

2.3.51

SIDE

BAND: Spread the band width over your L ear. Your R hand will hold one end of the band in front of your face, and the L hand will hold the other end of the band behind your head. (2.3.51)

    a. Push the head to the L side, leading with your L ear.

    b. Change the band and repeat on the R side.

2. STRETCH WITH MORE RESISTANCE

DIAGONAL

BAND: Put the band on the back of your head.

    a. Rotate your torso and lower your head to the opposite knee. (2.3.52)

    b. Lift your head against your pull on the band.

    c. Change the band and repeat on the second side.

BACK OF THE NECK STRETCH

BAND: Wrap the band along the back of the head.

    a. Bend your head forward.

    b. Slowly and gently pull the band down and sustain this position while exerting very gentle pressure.

    c. Hold for one second, then release.

    d. Repeat on the second side

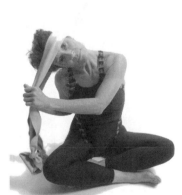

2.3.52

NOTE: For a more advanced stretch, try to release a little while applying the gentle pressure and then allow the head to sink lower with gravity again (P.N.F.).

SIDE STRETCH

BAND: Lower the R ear down towards the R shoulder, with the nose and chin facing forward. Spread the band over your L ear from front to back as in #1: SIMPLE NECK. (2.3.53)

    a. Slowly and gently pull the band down toward the R side. Sustain this position while exerting very gentle pressure.

    b. Hold for one second, then release the resistance.

2.3.53

c. Rise to center (upright) with some resistance in the band.

d. Repeat a.–c. on the second side.

NOTE: For a more advanced stretch, try to release a little while applying the gentle pressure and then allow the head to sink lower with gravity again (P.N.F.).

Lessons from Life

#1. CHANGING HABITS

Losing weight—losing fat.

We know by now that our main goal for good health is to maintain a lean body. This does not necessarily mean losing weight, per se. It simply means that we should alter our fat-to-lean body ratio, so that the fat percentage is within a desirable range. It would be best to empty some of our fat cells and increase the muscle fibers. Even if the actual numbers on the scale do not change that much, our overall appearance will improve.

We also know in order to achieve this goal, we should eat a balance of foods that are low in fat content. We should also do physical activity at a low intensity (60–70%) of capacity for a relatively long duration (one hour) on a regular basis.

Since we know these facts, why is it hard for us to put this knowledge into practice? Why is it that every single time I pass my bathroom scale I step on it, looking for the results with anticipation, just as I have been doing for the last twenty years? The answer is one word: habit. Think of the habits you have acquired over your lifetime. Can you come up with one that you would like to change?

#2. MOVEMENT IS EVERYWHERE

There are many places where we can find movement if we look for it. When I was a child, I remember seeing a photograph of oil on a small pool of water. It was a color photo, so I could see the wonderful colors swirling with the motion of the water. Another place where I remember seeing movement was in the multicolored specks of the terrazzo tiles on our bathroom floor. When I used my imagination, I saw connections between the different colored patterns, and I made the shapes into a story.

#3. SKY MOVEMENT

One of my favorite places of movement is the clouds. I used to walk home from school with my head back, gazing up at them, watching them sail past. They became animals, historic figures, or characters from mysterious stories, depending on how the wind blew them. Now, thirty years later, I still watch them when I lie back in my hammock or in the Jacuzzi. The movement up in the sky is still going on.

#4. WALKING PEOPLE, MOVING PARTS

During the last year of my army service, I was stationed at a remote little kibbutz out in the Israeli desert. It was really a very harsh transition when I decided to leave the kibbutz and move to the crowded city of Tel Aviv. Once I got there, I remember seeing people everywhere I looked. I developed a great fear of crowds because I was not used to so many people around me at one time. The main street in Tel Aviv, Dizengoff Street, was the busiest of all. It was also the street I had to walk through every day to get to my apartment. I tried to shield myself from my fear by concentrating on just a specific part of every one around me. For example, as I passed through the street on any given day, I might see only eyes; on another day, it might be lips, or shoulder movements, or the tops of heads, and so on. I found that if I separated the people into smaller parts, I could cope with them. This proved to be a very effective way to deal with a pavement full of walking people.

#5. HEALING COMES FIRST

I had a dance student come to me one morning to talk. She told me about a disturbing incident she had experienced in the past and how it had affected her life, her dreams, and her relationships. Her nervous system was filled with emotion. Her cry carried through her whole body. All I could do for her at that moment was to put my hand firmly on her sternum to allow her to bring herself to awareness and to give her the time and space she needed. Dance and movement were her means of release and escape, but she could not pursue them until she worked out this other major issue. She dropped out of the dance program, knowing that she could not truly do it well until she had worked through her past and healed.

#6. ENDLESS POSSIBILITIES

Imagine having a high-rise on the seashore. In the distance, you can see an open place. In that open space, your movement possibilities are endless. What would you choose to do?

#7. AUTHENTIC DANCE

Imagine taking a risk: Dance with your eyes closed, supporting the inner focus, diving into your own depth, finding your own body expressions (not just repeating movements you have already learned). Can you let your movement flow naturally, without projection, without interpretation, or without judgment? Can you trust yourself fully by stepping outside what you consider "safe"? That is being authentic.

#8. INNER AWARENESS

Awareness is one of the elements—along with physical and internal sensation, movement, thought, and feelings—that makes up our self-image. Awareness is how we know what we know about ourselves. One exercise to increase our own awareness is scanning the body. Lie down on the floor and imagine you are looking at yourself from the ceiling. Compare the two sides of your body. What do you see? Now draw your attention inward. Try to sense the spaces between your body and the floor and the points at which your body weight creates pressure against the floor. Now pay attention to the inner sensations of your bone, muscles, fluids, and organs. This process takes time. It is an internal "listening" to master. Give yourself at least twenty to thirty minutes each time you do this exercise in order to develop your skills. Do not become discouraged and give up halfway through. Allow yourself the time you need to create a new relationship within yourself.

#9. HURRICANES MOVE!

When the first edition of this book was going through its final "winding-up" stages, with the photographs being organized and assigned to the correct pages, a tremendous source of movement forced us to sit up and take notice of it: it was Hurricane Andrew. Besides the danger and destruction, it was really fascinating to watch the hurricane from above—the spiral movement of the clouds circling on the outskirts of the storm, the short-lived peace in the eye. However, the beauty of it ends once you find that you are caught in its raging path.

#10. SHRUGGING OFF ATLAS

Another way to relax those tired trapezius muscles at the top of your torso, on the days that you feel like Atlas with the whole sky resting on your shoulders: Shrug your shoulders up toward your ears, and hold them there as tensely as you can. You should begin to get a warm, shivering sensation. Hold them there for a while; then simply let them drop to their normal position as you exhale. Although it seems that tensing the shoulder muscles will only make them feel worse, they actually will feel freer and more relaxed.

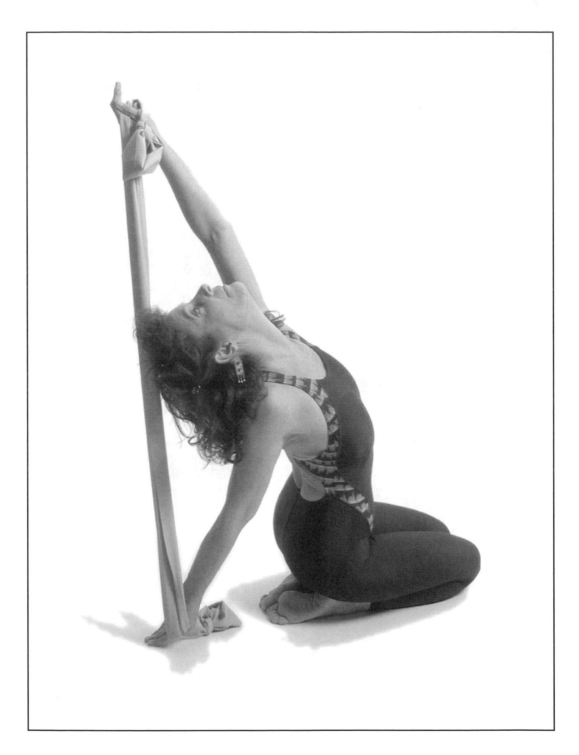

Chapter 2
Chapter Two: Exercises

PART 4: WARM-UP CLOSURE

Every man is the builder of a temple, called his body, to the God he worships, after a style purely his own, nor can he get off by hammering marble instead. We are all sculptors and painters, and our material is our own flesh and blood and bones. Any nobleness begins at once to refine a man's features, any meanness to imbrute them.

— Henry David Thoreau
Walden and Other Writings (1993: 185)

MUSCLES OF THE POSTERIOR TORSO

1. Erector spinae
2. Spinalis dorsi
3. Semispinalis cervicis (2.4.1)
4. Semispinalis capitis (2.4.2)

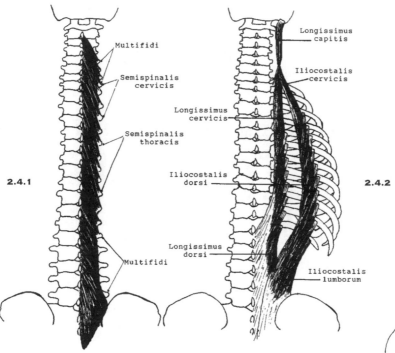

5. Longissimus dorsi (2.4.2)
6. Longissimus cervicis (2.4.2)
7. Longissimus capitis (2.4.2 and 2.4.8)
8. Iliocostalis lumborum (2.4.2)
9. Iliocostalis dorsi (2.4.2)
10. Iliocostalis cervicis (2.4.2)
11. Splenius capitis (2.4.3)
12. Splenius cervicis (2.4.3)

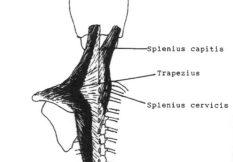

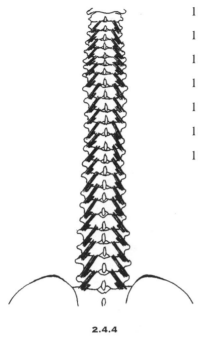

2.4.4

13. Rotators of the entire spinal column (2.4.4)

14. Multifidi of the entire spinal column (2.4.1)

15. Suboccipital

16. Serratus superior

17. Serratus inferior

18. Interspinales of the entire spinal column

19. Intertransversarii of the entire spinal column

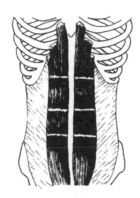

2.4.5

MUSCLES OF THE ANTERIOR TORSO

1. Rectus abdominis (2.4.5)

2. Obliquus externus abdominis (2.4.6)

3. Obliquus internus abdominis (2.4.7)

4. Transversus abdominis

5. External intercostal

6. Internal intercostal

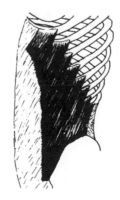

2.4.6

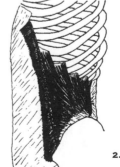

2.4.7

MUSCLES OF THE HEAD AND NECK

1. Longus colli
2. Longus capitis
3. Rectus capitis anterior
4. Rectus capitis lateralis
5. Rectus capitis major (2.4.8)
6. Rectus capitis minor (2.4.8)

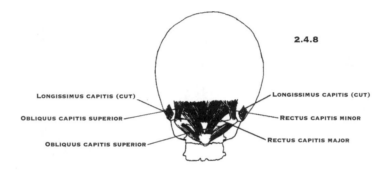

2.4.8

7. Scalenus anterior (2.4.9)
8. Scalenus medius (2.4.9)
9. Scalenus posterior (2.4.9)
10. Splenius capitis (2.4.3)
11. Splenius cervicis (2.4.3)
12. Obliquus capitis inferior (2.4.8)
13. Obliquus capitis superior (2.4.8)
14. Trapezius (2.4.9)

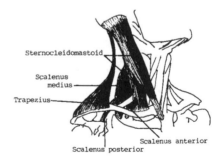

2.4.9

I. P.N.F.: THE INFINITY SYMBOL: ∞

(VIDEO VOLUME I: CENTER OF BODY, VII)

NOTE: The following exercise is based on the Proprioceptive Neurological Facilitation (PNF) in physical therapy. It was developed by the neurophysiologist Herman Kabat, M.D., Ph.D., who believed that diagonal and spiral paths are inherent in the organizational structure of muscular architecture and use.

POSITION:

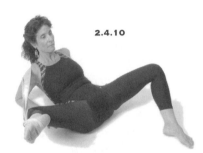

2.4.10

a. Sit down and bend both knees, so that the soles of the feet are flat on the floor and the legs are parallel to each other.

- Both knees should point toward the ceiling.

b. Lean slightly backward, supporting your body weight behind you with your forearms on the floor.

- Both elbows should be bent.

- The arms are parallel with the fingers near your pelvis.

- Keep the torso elevated; do not let your shoulders shrug or the body relax.

BAND: Attach one end of the band to your R foot. Stretch the remainder of the band across your R shoulder, behind your back, and down your L arm. Hold it in your L hand. Wrap the band once around the L hand, and hold it on the floor to stabilize it.

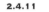

2.4.11

EXERCISE:

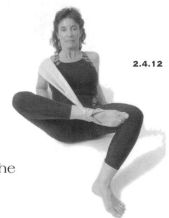

2.4.12

a. With both hips on the floor, open the R leg 45° to the side and diagonally upward off the floor. (2.4.10)

- The band is stretched as the leg is extended and slackens as the knee bends.

b. Think of tracing a horizontal figure eight (the symbol for infinity: ∞) between the stationary knee and the diagonal, leading with the big toe. (2.4.11, 2.4.12, and 2.4.13)

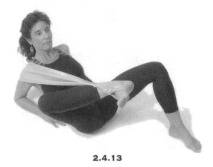

2.4.13

- Both hips stay on the floor throughout the entire exercise, but the upper body and head will move with the movement.
- This is more about body integration than about stretching the band.

c. Repeat tracing the infinity sign the number of times your program requires.

d. Repeat b.–c., tracing the figure eight by leading with the little toe toward the knee and out to the diagonal, instead of the big toe. (2.4.14 and 2.4.15)

e. Change the band and repeat a.–d. on the second side.

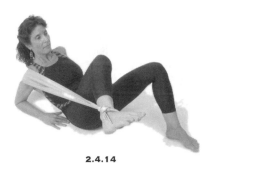

2.4.14

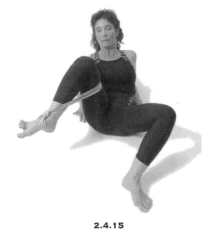

2.4.15

II. HALF-MOON TWIST

(VIDEO VOLUME I: CENTER OF BODY, VIII)

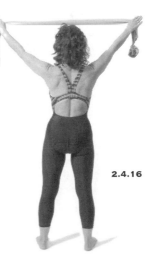

2.4.16

POSITION:

1. Stand in a parallel position with your legs hips-width apart.

2. Slightly bend the knees.

3. Place the arms overhead in a V-shape.

BAND: Hold one end of the band in each hand, at a place on the band that allows your arms to make the V-shape while stretching the band a little. (2.4.16)

- When you stand, the ends of the band will hand down on each side of your arms.

EXERCISE:

1. SIMPLE

a. Bend your torso and upper body laterally (sidewise) to the L side, stretching both arms to each side until they are at shoulder level. (2.4.17)

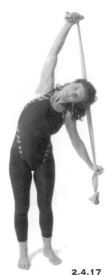

2.4.17

- Head drops to the L, face facing forward.
- The band stretches behind the head, almost resting on the shoulders.
- Keep the hips centered. Bend as far over to the side as you can without allowing the R hip to shift out of alignment.

b. While you are still bent over to the side, rotate the torso from the waist one quarter of a turn to the L side, as if you are trying to look at the floor.

c. Rotate back again to the lateral bend to the side, torso facing forward.

d. Slowly straighten the body back to the original upright position by initiating the torso lift from the upper arm.

- Roll the body up one vertebra at a time.
- The abdominal muscles should support the back muscles.

e. Repeat a.–d. on the second side.

127

2. SIMPLE, WITH BENT LEGS (not on video)

  a. Repeat #1: SIMPLE, above, with the knees bent.

    • Have your head face down or up to work different muscle groups in your neck and shoulders. (2.4.18)

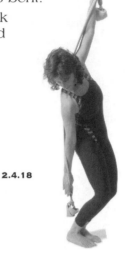

2.4.18

III. LATERALS

(VIDEO VOLUME I: CENTER OF BODY, IX)

POSITION: Sit with the legs in a wide, turned-out second position (straddle split), as far to each side as is comfortable. The torso is upright and the arms are held over the head, shoulder-width apart.

BAND: Hold the band in both hands comfortably, neither stretched nor loose. (2.4.19)

EXERCISES:

1. ISOLATED SIDE REACH

ONE ARM

2.4.19

  a. Isolate the R arm, and open it to the R side. (2.4.20)

  b. Return to the starting position.

FROM THE HIP JOINT

  a. Repeat #1: ISOLATED SIDE REACH, ONE ARM, above, adding the torso moving from the L hip joint as you reach.

    • This is a small movement.

RIBS LEAD

  a. Shift the body to the R side by leading with the R ribs.

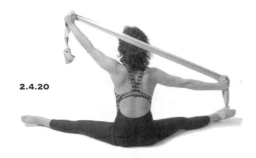

2.4.20

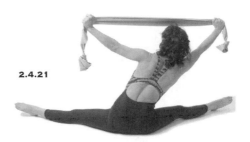

2.4.21

- The R arm will reach out and up on a diagonal, as the ONE ARM reach, but only to the point where you are still sitting on both hips. (2.4.21)
- Leave the L arm where it is.
- This is a bigger movement than FROM THE HIP JOINT, above.

b. Return to starting position.

SECOND SIDE: Repeat all parts of #1: ISOLATED SIDE REACH to the L.

2. SIDE CURVE

a. Curve your upper body over to the R side, initiating the movement from the head and moving down through your verte-bras. (2.4.22)

b. Stretch each side of the band toward shoulder level as you bend.

2.4.22

- The R arm will open diagonally downward, and the L arm will stretch diagonally upward.

c. Return to starting position by lifting up, rib-by-rib.

d. Repeat a.–c. on the second side.

3. SIDE CURVE TWIST

a. Bend the body laterally to the R as in #2: SIDE CURVE, above. (2.4.22)

b. At the depth of your bend, pull your R hip back and rotate the torso down to face the leg. (2.4.23, next page)

c. Untwist by using your opposite hip and abdominal muscles to initi-ate the return of the torso to the lateral bend directly side.

d. Lift your torso to return to the upright position.

e. Repeat a.–d. on the second side.

129

4. VARIATIONS:

You may repeat #1.–3. with your legs in different positions: a narrow sitting second position, a parallel first position, or cross-legged.

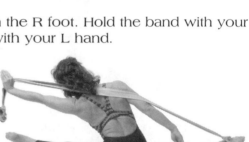

- All shifts and bends move to "true side," not over your leg.

5. ADVANCED LATERALS (not on video)

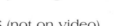
2.4.23

STARTING POSITION:

a. Sit with both legs wide in a second position, as far apart as possible.

- Keep the knees facing up toward the ceiling.

b. Adjust the band in your hand so that it will provide you with the right amount of resistance.

BAND: Place one end of the band on the R foot. Hold the band with your R hand. For more of a workout, hold it with your L hand.

EXERCISES:

BODY SHIFT

a. Shift the body, so the torso and arm stretch up on a diagonal to the L side. (2.4.24)

- The torso does not bend.

b. Hold this position for a few seconds.

c. Return to the starting position.

d. Repeat according to your workout program.

2.4.24

BODY BENDS

a. Bend your body laterally to the L side, so that your face and body are forward.

- You will be bending directly sidewise and not diagonally over your leg.

b. At the depth of your bend, turn your face and body down as if you were looking at the floor under your face. (2.4.25)

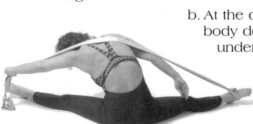

c. The right side of your hip and abdominals rotate the body back to the lateral bend (i.e., untwist).

d. Lift the body up to the starting position.

2.4.25

SECOND SIDE: Change the band and repeat #5: ADVANCED LATERALS on the second side.

6. COMBINATION
   a. Create a smooth combination of the #5: ADVANCED LATERALS: BODY SHIFTS and BODY BENDS.

IV. THE BODY BUILDER

(VIDEO VOLUME I: CENTER OF BODY, X)

POSITION: Lie on the floor on your back with your legs parallel, about hips-width apart. Bend the legs, facing both knees up toward the ceiling.
   • The soles of the feet are flat on the floor.
   • The pelvis is in "neutral" so that your back neither arches nor flattens.
BAND:
   a. Place one end of the band on each foot.
   b. The remainder of the band runs along the outside of the ankle and is held in each hand at navel height. (2.4.26)

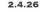

   c. Hold both arms about chest-width apart with the elbows straight, but not hyperextended.

2.4.26

   d. Once you are in position, the band will be held directly above your navel.

EXERCISES:

1. SIMPLE
   a. Bring the arms directly overhead and down toward the floor (over your head) as much as you can. (2.4.27)
      • Do not arch your back.
      • Exhale on the lift.

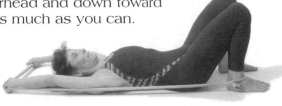

2.4.27

b. Reverse the action to return the arms slowly to the starting position again.

• Exhale on the return.

2. CROSS-BODY

STARTING POSITION: With one loop on the L foot, take the loop off the R foot and hold the band over your navel with the R hand alone. The L arm is on the floor at your side, with the palm facing down in order to stabilize yourself and help keep your balance.

• In this exercise, the L foot and R arm work together.

a. Extend the L leg and R arm 90° up toward the ceiling.

b. Lower the straight leg to the floor below you by pulling the leg out of the hip joint, creating a large arc. At the same time, stretch the R arm and the band overhead to the floor. (2.4.28)

c. Slowly, return to the beginning position by reversing the movements.

• Exhale on the stretch away and exhale again on the return.

d. Change the band and repeat a.–c. on the second side.

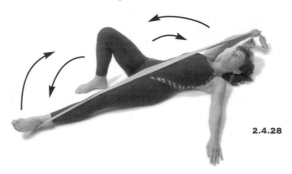

2.4.28

3. ONE SIDE (not on video):

STARTING POSITION: Hold the band with the L hand with one loop on the L foot.

1. Repeat #2: CROSS BODY, with this new position. (2.4.29)

NOTE: You will be working the same arm and leg, instead of working in opposition as you did in #2: CROSS BODY.

2.4.29

4. BOTH ARMS AND LEGS EXTENSION

STARTING POSITION: Same as the starting position described

at the beginning of V. THE BODY BUILDER. Hold the band with both hands directly in front of you.

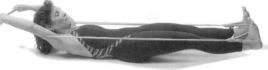

NOTE: In this exercise, both arms and both legs work together at the same time. Start and finish simultaneously.

2.4.30

a. Extend both arms and legs straight up into the air.

• Palms may face up or down.

b. Reach the arms to the floor overhead at the same time as the legs move in a large arc to the floor below you. (2.4.30)

• You may only be able to move part of the way to the floor at first.

c. Slowly, return to the beginning position by reversing the movements.

• As you become stronger, you will move all the way to the floor. (2.4.31)

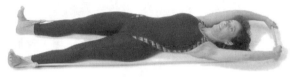

2.4.31

V. THE ARCHER'S BOW

(VIDEO VOLUME I: CENTER OF BODY, XI)

POSITION: Lie on your stomach (in a prone position) with your face down. Extend your arms overhead. Extend your legs on the floor.

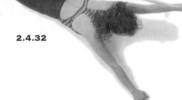

BAND: Attach one end of the band to the R foot. Hold the other end in the L hand at a point on the band that will give you the right amount of resistance. (2.4.32)

• The band will be across your back.

• Exhale on each lift and lowering.

2.4.32

EXERCISES:

NOTE: Be sure to lengthen the limbs from their sockets before lifting them.

133

1. CROSS BODY

NOTE: Instead of this order, you may do ONE ARM, ONE LEG, and then ARM AND LEG together.

ARM AND LEG

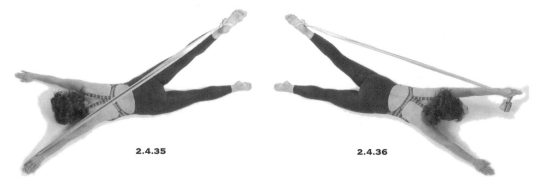

2.4.33

a. Simultaneously, lift the L arm and the R leg off the floor.

- Allow the upper body to lift and look to the horizon. (2.4.33)

- Hand and foot move to the same level. Do not lift one more than the other.

- Exhale on the lifting and on the lowering.

b. Extend and return slowly to the floor again.

ONE ARM

2.4.34

a. With the band stretched in the starting position, isolate and lift the L arm only. (2.4.34)

b. Extend and slowly return to the floor again.

- Allow the L side of the body to lift as the eyes follow the hand.

ONE LEG (not on video)

a. With the band stretched in the starting position, isolate and lift the R leg only. (2.4.35)

b. Slowly return to the floor again.

- Both hips stay on the floor.

- It may be easier to turn your face to the side of the working leg.

SECOND SIDE: Change the band and repeat on the second side.

2.4.35

2.4.36

2. ARM AND LEG, SAME SIDE

STARTING POSITION: Attach the ends of the band to the L leg and the L hand, so you are working the same side of the body. (2.4.36)

    a. Repeat all four #1: CROSS BODY exercises above on both sides.

    3. REST: Roll to your back and rest with your arms hugging your bent knees, which are on your chest.

VI. DEEP ROTATION OF THE BACK (ADVANCED)

(VIDEO VOLUME I: CENTER OF BODY, XII)

POSITION: Lie on your stomach (in a prone position) with your face down. Extend your arms overhead in either a V-shape (as seen in 2.4.32) or with both arms bent and directly above your head (as on the video). Extend your legs on the floor.

BAND: Attach one end of the band to the R foot. Run the remainder of the band along the R side of the back. If your arms are in a V-shape as in the photograph, run it over the L shoulder, and then hold it with your L hand at a point on the band that will give you the right amount of resistance. If both hands are together, as in the video, hold the band in both hands above your head and on the floor.

EXERCISE:

    a. Flex the L foot and turn the toes down into the floor.
       • Use the L foot and the forehead as anchors for your balance.
       • Bend the L knee slightly, if needed.
    b. Lengthen the R leg and lift it up behind you as high as it is comfortable, keeping the leg straight and foot, pointed. (2.4.37)

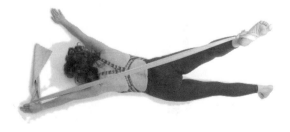

2.4.37

135

c. At the highest point, bend the R leg into a back (derrière) attitude position and shorten the band. (2.3.38)

d. Move the R leg (in attitude position) across the L leg. Try to touch the floor with the toes of the R foot on the other side of the L leg, reaching over as far as you can. (2.4.39)

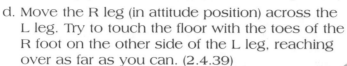

- You might not touch the floor if it is too great a stretch.
- Your whole torso will spiral in response to the leg movement.

2.4.38

- Work very slowly, with control.

e. As you return, initiate the movement from your pelvis, lifting the R foot and knee as high as possible.

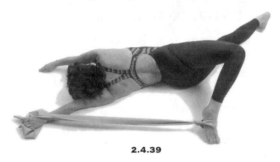

2.4.39

f. Return to the starting position by rotating the hip back to center, as the leg follows and reverses its movement in the largest arc possible.

g. SECOND SIDE: Change the band and repeat on the second side.

h. Roll to your back, hug your knees to your chest, and rest.

VII. DEEP ROTATION OF THE UPPER TORSO (ADVANCED)

(VIDEO VOLUME I: CENTER OF BODY, XIII)

POSITION:

a. Lie on your L side with both legs bent comfortably in front of the body; knee on top of knee, foot on top of foot.

b. Straighten the arms on the floor directly in front of the shoulders, and have the elbows softened slightly. (2.4.40)

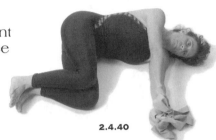

2.4.40

BAND: To get the proper length for the band, hold it a little wider apart than shoulder-width. Then put both hands together.

EXERCISE:

NOTE: The goal is to spiral the back, resisting the tendency for the lower back to join the action. Think of keeping the lower and middle back erect despite the rotation of the upper torso.

a. Inhale as you lengthen and lift the R arm up toward the ceiling, creating a large arc.

b. Exhale as you keep your arm at shoulder height: allow your head, eyes, neck, and back to rotate with the moving arm and continue to the other side toward the floor. (2.4.41)

• The upper back will spiral. The pelvis and legs remain fixed.

c. As you return to the beginning position, lengthen your arm away from your body and return with the biggest arc you can create.

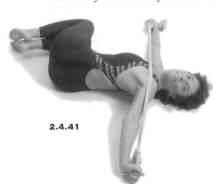

2.4.41

• Work slowly, and exhale as you rotate in each direction.

d. Change your position and the band, and repeat a.–d. on the second side.

e. Roll to your back and hug your knees to rest.

VIII. PEARL NECKLACE

(VIDEO VOLUME I: CENTER OF BODY, XIV)

POSITION: Sit on your knees or on the edge of a chair. Hold your arms overhead, slightly wider than shoulder-width apart.

BAND: Hold the band in both hands.

EXERCISES:

NOTE: Throughout the exercises in this section, think of each of the vertebras in your spine as an individual pearl on a necklace. As you curve your spine, each one is affected in progression.

2.4.42

1. SIMPLE

   a. Lower your arms to shoulder height, stretching the band behind your head. (2.4.42 shows just the arm movement.)

   b. At the same time, allow the head to roll downward to the front, curving your tailbone inward and tilting your pelvis backward. (2.4.43 shows the scoop before the arms have moved.)

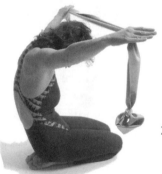

      • This is like the scoop in I. THE ICE CREAM SCOOPER on pg. 43.

      • This will lengthen your spine into a "C" shape.

   c. Return by initiating the movement from the tailbone, and roll the spine back to the original position one vertebra at a time.

2. SIMPLE, VARIATION (not on video)

   a. Repeat #1: SIMPLE, above, but return by initiating the movement of the spine from the head rather than the tailbone.

2.4.43

3. TORSO ROTATION

   a. As in SIMPLE, above, tilt the pelvis backward and roll the head forward, creating a "C" shape in your spine.

   b. Lower your arms and the band to shoulder height.

   c. While you are in that position, rotate the torso to the R side without changing the relationship between the arms and the body. (2.4.44)

      • Exhale with this movement.

d. Rotate back to the center and roll the spine back to the original position one vertebra at a time.

- You may do this by initiating the movement either from the tailbone or from the head.

e. Repeat a.–d. on the second side.

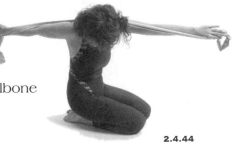

2.4.44

4. WITH HIGH RELEASE

a. Start as in #3: TORSO ROTATION.

b. Once you curve the spine into a "C" shape and rotate to the R side, continue by leading with the R arm diagonally to the floor behind you and the L arm diagonally upward in front of your body and toward the ceiling.

- You will finish with your body in a high release, bending up and back. Your L arm reaches directly up and you look down toward the floor.

c. Change the focus of your eyes and head upward to your L arm. (2.4.45)

d. Reach upward, from the L arm, using your abdominal muscles to lift and support the hyperextended back into a sitting position.

- L arm reaches up.
- Face faces forward with your torso turned to the R side. (2.4.46)

2.4.45　　e. Rotate the torso to face center, in the same direction as your knees.

f. Bring your arms overhead to the starting position.

g. Repeat a.–f. on the second side.

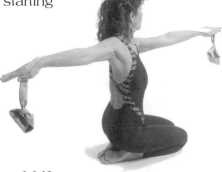

2.4.46

IX. WORKING WITH A BARRE

NOTE:

- In each of the exercises in this section, you will need a ballet barre. If you do not have access to a barre, other objects may be used instead: a doorknob, the edge of a *sturdy* piece of furniture, a strong towel rack, or a railing.

- These exercises are a special feature of this book and are not demonstrated on the *Get Stronger by Stretching with Thera-Band®* video.

POSITION: Please note the body and band positions in the individual exercises.

BAND: Wrap the center of the band over the barre once or twice. The ends of the band will hang down.

EXERCISES:

1. LEGS, ON YOUR BACK

STARTING POSITION

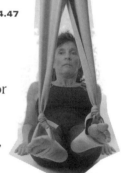

2.4.47

    a. Attach the ends of the band to each foot.

    b. Lie on your back with your lower body on the floor and your upper body supported by your lower arms.

    c. Shift your body slightly back, away from the barre, to create tension in the band. (2.4.47)

      • Your feet are raised a little off the floor.

EXERCISE

    a. Lower both legs toward the floor. (2.4.48)

    b. Return slowly.

2.4.48

    c. Repeat as your program requires.

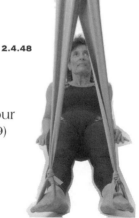

2. LEGS, ON YOUR STOMACH

STARTING POSITION: Keep the band wrapped on your feet as you turn your body over to lie face down. (2.4.49)

    EXERCISE

    a. Lower both legs toward the floor. (2.4.50)

    b. Return slowly.

    c. Repeat as your program requires.

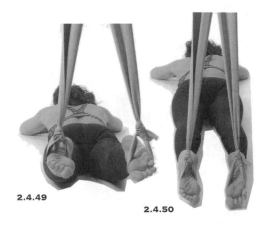

2.4.49

2.4.50

3. ARMS, ON YOUR STOMACH

STARTING POSITION:

    a. Remain on your stomach, below the barre.

    b. Hold one band loop in each hand.

    c. Shift your body away from the barre to create tension in the lifted arms. (2.4.51)

    d. Lift your head and upper torso slightly off the floor.

EXERCISE

    a. Lower both arms toward the floor. (2.4.52)

    b. Return slowly.

    c. Repeat as your program requires.

4. ARMS, ON YOUR BACK

STARTING POSITION

    a. Turn your body, so that you are on your back, below the barre (in a supine position).

    b. Hold one band loop in each hand.

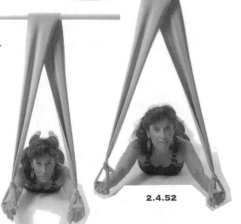

2.4.52

2.4.51

    c. Shift your body away from the barre to create tension in the lifted arms.

      • Your head and upper torso stay on the floor.

EXERCISE

    a. Lower both arms toward the floor. (2.4.53)

    b. Return slowly.

    c. Repeat as your program requires.

5. LEGS, ON YOUR SIDE

STARTING POSITION:

    a. Lie on your R side with bottom leg bent and top leg extended. (2.4.54, next page)

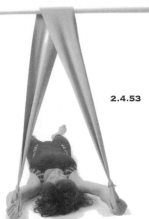

2.4.53

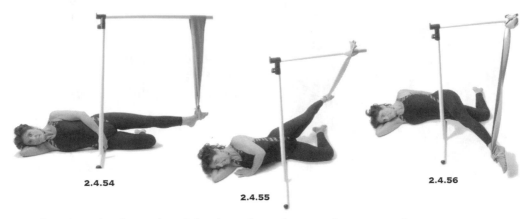

2.4.54

2.4.55

2.4.56

b. Wrap both ends of the band on the top foot. In order to create tension in the band, shift the body forward, so you are underneath the barre.

EXERCISE:

a. Lower the top leg to the floor.

b. Return to the starting position.

c. Repeat as your program requires.

d. Change your body position and band and repeat a.–c. on the second side.

6. SWING

STARTING POSITION: As #5: LEGS, ON YOUR SIDE, above, except wrap one end of the band around the ankle, and the other end around the arch of the foot. Flex or point the top foot.

EXERCISE:

a. Swing the top leg gently backward and forward. (2.4.55 and 2.4.56)

b. Repeat as your program requires.

c. Change your body position and band and repeat a.–c. on the second side.

7. OPEN/CLOSE

STARTING POSITION:

a. Sit facing the barre with the ends of the band on your ankles or feet.

b. Extend your legs in front of you. (2.4.57)

c. Shift your body back slightly to create tension, but keep your heels on the floor.

2.4.57

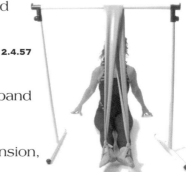

142

d. Support your upper body with your fingers on the floor diagonally behind you and bend your elbows.
  - Keep the abdominal muscles working against the back.
  - Keep the torso straightened and lifted, not sunk back into the body.
  - Shoulders are pressed down.

EXERCISE:

a. Open your legs slowly to a wide second position. (2.4.58)

b. Close your legs again, being sure your heels stay on the floor.

c. Repeat as your program requires.

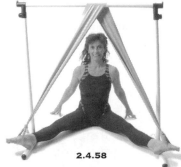

2.4.58

8. SPIRAL/ARM

STARTING POSITION:

a. Sit facing the barre, far enough away so that you can extend both arms directly in front of you and touch the barre.

b. Hold one end of the band with the R hand while you stabilize the other end on the barre with the L hand. (2.4.59)

EXERCISE:

a. Extend the R arm to the side and behind you on a diagonal, turning the upper body and head as you turn. (2.4.60)

b. Return slowly to the starting position.

c. Repeat as your program requires.

d. Change your body position and band and repeat a.–c. on the second side.

2.4.59   2.4.60   2.4.61

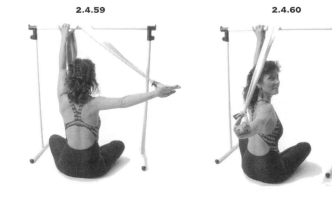
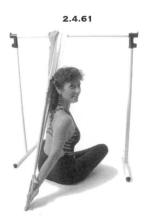

9. SPIRAL/ARM LOWERS

a. Repeat SPIRAL, ARM on page 143, pressing your extended arm to the floor after you rotate it behind you, and lifting it back up. (2.4.61)

10. LEG ROTATION:

STARTING POSITION:

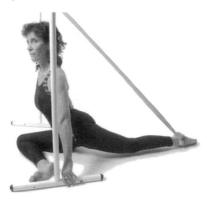

2.4.62

a. Sit in fourth position underneath the barre, with the R leg in front of your body and the L leg behind you as far as possible. (2.4.62)

b. Place both ends of the band on your L foot.

EXERCISE:

a. Lift the L foot off the floor by inwardly rotating the whole leg in the hip socket.

b. Lower the L foot down toward the ground by outwardly rotating the whole leg in the hip socket.

• This is a variation on THE LITTLE MERMAID'S TAIL on page 79.

11. LEG EXTENSION:

STARTING POSITION: Sit in the same position as in LEG ROTATION, above. (2.4.62)

EXERCISE:

a. Extend the L leg directly behind you in an arabesque aligned behind the L side of your back. (2.4.63)

b. Return by releasing the knee into the floor and bending the lower leg back into the fourth position.

2.4.63

Lessons from Life

#1. AMERICA, A SURPRISE

I came to America in 1982 with strong idealism about what would create a fit body: adequate sleep, good nutrition, healthy relationships, comfort, natural fabrics, and soft shoes. These were all in addition to basics: a good balance between flexibility and strength, acrobic fitness and endurance, and efficiency of movement and grace. However, as I was adjusting to my new life here in America I watched television and spoke with people. The picture that I got of what Americans thought about their health was quite different. Gyms offer "life-time memberships" where you could learn how to focus on isolating specific muscles and to strengthen them on machines, rather than learning how to integrate all of them in movement. I also saw how people repeatedly danced to rock and roll music in a way that is too hard on their joints in order to make their hearts race. Needless to say, I was surprised and a little disappointed.

#2. BACKS AND INFANTS

People put a lot of thought and energy into making lives easier for themselves, disengaging themselves from things with "ease" in mind. For example, a mother is busy, and she cannot get anything done because the baby needs to be touched and carried all the time. The mother takes the child who can not sit, crawl, or walk yet, and puts him or her in a "walker," a rolling chair that keeps his back supported in a sitting position, so he or she can keep up with her. Do people think they can outsmart nature? Do we really believe that a child will have a strong enough back to carry him through life when he is made to skip the necessary developmental stages on the floor? Is it any wonder people miss many days from work each year because of back problems?

#3. RELAXATION

At times, the days seem short and the schedule is full of things that need to be done. One of the ways I cope with the stresses in my life is by doing a relaxation technique. It takes only five to ten minutes, but makes me feel rejuvenated once again. Lie down. Bring both knees up to your chest, legs about hip-width apart. Let them drop down directly below you so the soles of your feet are on the floor and your knees are pointing up to the ceiling. If you feel pressure behind your lower back, you may put some support under your backside (gluteus muscles) so that the pelvis rotates slightly backward. You may use a towel, pair of socks, small pillow, or even your own hand (open or in a fist).

Close your eyes and focus inward. Visualize the space inside of your body entirely filled with sand or some kind of thick, slow-moving liquid, such as honey. Imagine little holes at certain places on the back side of your body—in the back of your skull, on each shoulder blade, on the pelvis (at each side of your spine), on the palms of your hands, and on the heels. Imagine the thick and heavy substance inside your body very slowly draining our of these holes and through the floor, just like grains of sand drain our of an hourglass. Once you find that you are "empty," you will be rested and ready to continue your busy day.

#4. EMOTIONAL MOVEMENT

Through years of being a muscle therapist, I have grown to recognize movement in areas other than in physical bodies. Relationships also are constantly changing and dynamic. Traumatic emotional experiences can cause injuries to a person just as surely as the physical ones can. The similarity goes even farther. If the trauma was severe enough, the person may also need the help of a different kind of therapist in order to heal. Most of the time, though, the disturbances that temporarily alter our balance are minor ones. Still, the way we choose to compensate for them may not be the most efficient way to handle the situation. In that case, it would be good to check our own emotional "alignment" every so often, to be certain that it can "support" us once again. I have found that, for myself, one of my own personality traits is to push forward too strongly in my relationships. Sometimes, especially at the most important times, I have found that doing this did not serve me well at all. I am learning to let go a little, to stop forcing the issue as much, and I am pleasantly surprised to discover this change is creating a vacuum; a space for new movement and new rhythm to the relationship. For me, this new pattern I have chosen allows me to "move more easily" through some of my relationships.

#5. NATURAL MOVEMENT

I believe that as we grow up, we give up movement. We limit our possibilities. For example, look at our shoes. We wear shoes that will shape our feet, not shoes in the shape of our feet. It is the same thing with our clothing. In addition, some people will sit for hours in chairs and not move. They always sit at the same height and at the same angle. Are we designed for stationary positions or for activity? Are we really using the muscle possibility that nature gave us?

#6. POSTURE, MOVEMENT PATTERNS

How many people do you know who rub the back of their neck with their hands while talking to you or who would really enjoy a good neck massage? How many are in pain? There is a direct correlation between improper posture and the biomechanics that cause a person's pain. In addition, dysfunctional movement patterns can cause physical pathological reflex arcs in the nervous system and can also increase the intrajoint pressure in the facet joints of the vertebral column. This is why incorrect posture can give you a real pain in the neck!

#7. MOVEMENT FREEDOM

In the summer of 1972, we were a group of teenagers who had just graduated from high school and who would soon be drafted into the Israeli army for two years of mandatory military service. We were willing to serve the country that wc grew up in, but we also had mixed feelings. There was fear and doubt about the way the occupied territories were being dealt with. There were just a few days left before we would be drafted, so we decided to have a big party. We cut the boys' long hair (which was very symbolic in those days), and then we drove south to the Sinai desert seashore. There was a giant sand dune of dry, white sand that had all of its wrinkles smoothly ironed out by the wind. We climbed up one side to the top of it, looking out over the beach. Then, we shed our clothes and rolled all the way down the other side, leaving our own prints in the sand where it had once been perfectly smooth and empty. From the bottom of the sand dune, it was a short run to the water. What a sense of movement! What a sense of freedom!

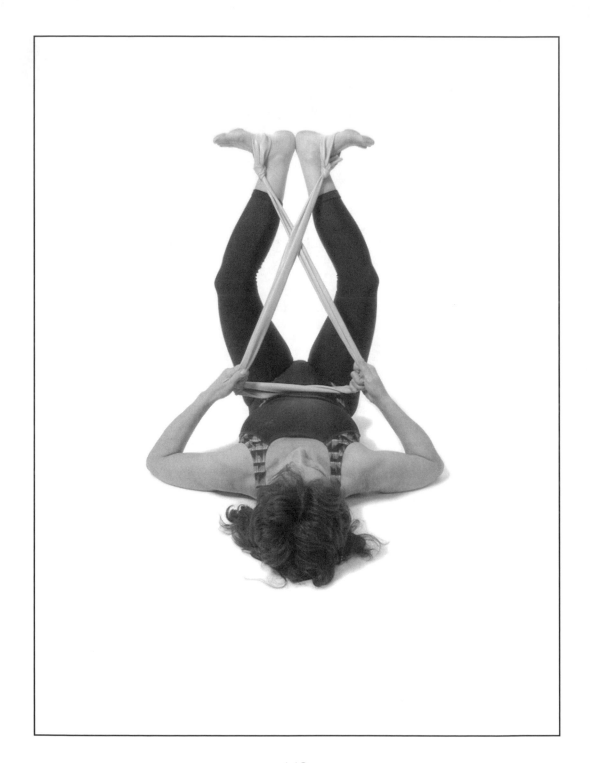

Chapter 2

Chapter Two: Exercises

PART 5: ESPECIALLY FOR DANCERS

Praise Him with the tambourine and dance!
Praise Him with stringed instruments and the pipe!
Praise Him with sounding cymbals!
Praise Him with loud clashing cymbals!
Let every thing that breathes praise the Lord!
Hallelujah!

—Psalm 150: 4–6

MUSCLES FOR OUTWARD ROTATION OF THE HIP

1. Gluteus medius (in hip adduction) (2.5.1)

2. Gluteus maximus (2.5.1)

3. The six deep lateral rotator muscles

   A. Piriformis (2.5.1)

   B. Superior gemellus (2.5.1)

   C. Obturator internus (2.5.1)

   D. Inferior gemellus (2.5.1)

   E. Obturator externus (2.5.1)

   F. Quadratus femoris (2.5.1)

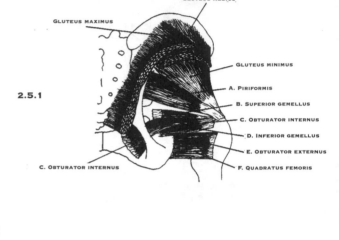

4. Iliopsoas (when thigh is flexed): psoas minor and psoas major (2.5.2)

5. Sartorius (when thigh is flexed) (2.5.2)

6. Biceps femoris (2.5.2)

7. Adductor brevis (in hip adduction) (2.5.2)

8. Adductor magnus (in hip adduction) (2.5.2)

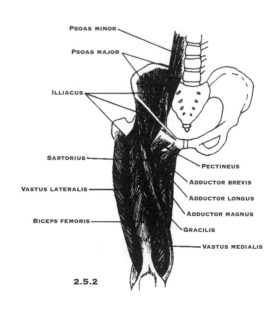

I. PREPARATION FOR ALLEGRO WORK

POSITION: Lie on your back with your legs at a 90° angle from the torso, with the soles of the feet flexed toward the ceiling. (An alternative position would be to sit in a parallel first position; see Appendix C.)

BAND: Either place one end of the band on each feet, or place the center of the band under the feet. When you have gotten into position, cross the band and hold the center of it in front of your chest or the loops. Hands are shoulder-width apart. (2.5.3)

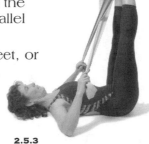

2.5.3

EXERCISES:

NOTE: Numbers 1–5 are similar to the exercises under Part 2: LOWER BODY: I ANTIGRAVITY LEG WORK, on page 61 but are included here again specifically as a preparation for jumps. When requested, do the exercises with *more energy and force*.

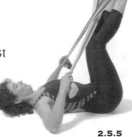

2.5.4

REPEAT all segments of PREPARATION FOR ALLEGRO WORK 4–8 times.

1. TURN OUT AND TURN IN

   a. Turn your legs out (2.5.4), and then back to parallel (2.5.3).

2. BEND AND STRETCH, PARALLEL

   a. Bend your knees while your legs are in parallel, so that your toes are on an imaginary line directly above your navel. Imagine another line that goes from the heels to the tailbone. (2.5.5)

   • Do not let the legs lean toward the face.

   b. Straighten the legs by lengthening them behind the knees. Push out with the heels.

3. BEND AND STRETCH, TURNED OUT

   a. Turn your legs out, so that your feet are in first position.

   b. Bend your knees into a demi-plié, opening the knees toward the sides. (2.5.6)

   c. Straighten the legs by pushing the heels upward.

2.5.5

4. TENDU FROM PLIÉ, JUMP

   a. Demi-plié as in #3: BEND AND STRETCH, TURNED OUT. (2.5.6)

   b. When both legs are bent, straighten the R leg into a tendu on a diagonal to the R side with both feet still flexed.

   c. Return to the diamond shape (demi-plié).

   d. Straighten the legs by pushing upward with the heels.

   e. Repeat a.–d. to the other side.

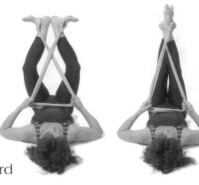

2.5.6   **2.5.7**

5. CHANGEMENT:

   a. Turn out the legs and place one foot in front of the other foot, in fifth position. (2.5.7)

   b. Open both legs a small distance to the side with the feet still flexed.

   c. Close to fifth position, changing which leg is in front. Gradually increase the tempo.

6. CHANGEMENT WITH WIDER OPENING

   a. Repeat #5: CHANGEMENT, above, opening your legs as wide as possible into second position on the "jumps." (2.5.8)

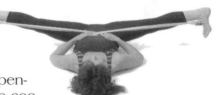
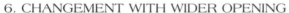

2.5.8

7. JUMPS IN PARALLEL SECOND

   a. Keeping the legs in parallel, open them a little wider than hip-width apart, in a parallel second position. (2.5.9)

   b. Bend the legs into a demi-plié.

   c. Push the legs forcefully up toward the ceiling.

8. JUMPS IN TURNED-OUT FIRST POSITION

   a. Repeat #7: JUMPS IN PARALLEL SECOND, except the legs are in a turned-out first position with the heels together. (2.5.10)

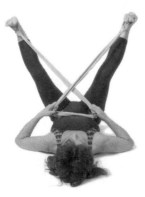

2.5.9

9. FOOT WORK, FIRST POSITION

a. Feet start in a parallel first position, feet flexed as much as possible. (2.5.3)

b. Point the feet with speed and force.

c. Repeat parts a.–c. of this exercise with the feet in a turned out first position. (2.5.4)

   • Work just with the feet.

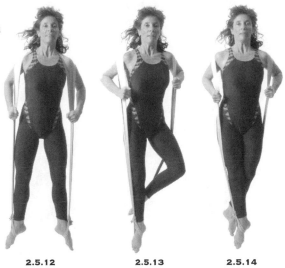

2.5.10

10. FOOT WORK, SECOND POSITION

a. Repeat #9: FOOT WORK, FIRST POSITION with feet in parallel second position (2.5.9) and turned-out second position. (2.5.11)

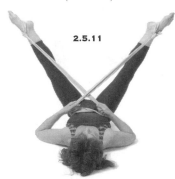

2.5.11

11. JUMPS IN FIRST AND SECOND POSITIONS

a. "Jump" up toward the ceiling, allowing your lower spine to lift off the floor.

   • Your upper back stays on the floor.

   • Combine the force and the speed of the legs with the force and the speed of the feet.

   • Complete this exercise in each of the positions in #9 and 10: parallel first, turned out first, parallel second, and turned out second

12. STANDING JUMPS

STARTING POSITION: Keep the ends of the bands attached to each foot and place the center of band over the shoulders and behind the head.

   • You will be using the band resistance as you actually jump (sauté).

EXERCISE:

a. Jump (sauté) in first and second positions—or any other jumping exercise that suits your needs. (2.5.12, 2.5.13, and 2.5.14)

2.5.12   2.5.13   2.5.14

II. ADVANCED BARRE WORK

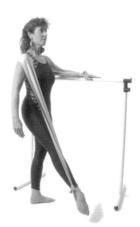

2.5.15

POSITION: Stand next to the barre, holding on to it with your L hand.

BAND: Attach one end of the band to the R foot. Spread the center of the band across the L shoulder. (2.5.15) The second loop will be held by the hand on the barre.

NOTE: Repeat all segments 4–8 times.

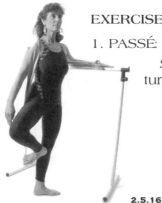

EXERCISE:

1. PASSÉ:

STARTING POSITION: Stand in a turned out first position.

a. Draw the flexed R foot up the R leg as high as you can without changing the level of your hip-bones. (2.5.16)

b. Return to standing.

c. Turn around, change the band, and repeat a.–b. with the L leg.

2.5.16

2. TENDU

a. From first position, tendu the flexed R foot devant (forward) with the heel going forward. (2.5.17)

b. Point the foot. (2.5.18 and 2.5.19)

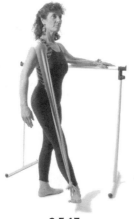

2.5.17

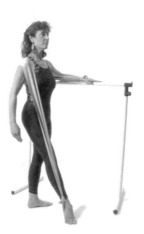

2.5.18

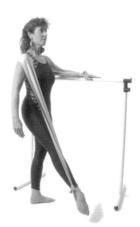

2.5.19

c. Close the foot again to first position, moving from the hip joint and pulling the toes back.

- Do the tendu very slowly, spreading the toes and going through demi-pointe each time.

d. Repeat en croix (front, side, back, and side).

e. Turn around, change the band, and repeat a.–d. with the L leg.

3. DÉGAGÉ

a. Repeat #2: TENDU, except the R foot will dégagé instead of tendu. (2.5.20)

4. ROND DE JAMBE:

a. With the foot flexed, rond de jambe the R leg on the floor (à terre) in any combination you are familiar with, both inward (en dedans) and outward (en dehors).

b. Repeat with the foot pointed.

c. Repeat a.–b. on the second side.

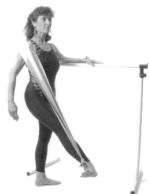

2.5. 20

5. ROND DE JAMBE EN L'AIR

a. Repeat #4: ROND DE JAMBE, except the rond de jambe will be in the air (en l'air).

6. FRAPPÉ

a. Use any frappé combination you are familiar with in an en croix pattern.

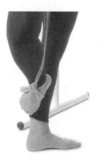

2.5.21

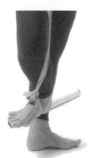

2.5. 22

- You may either do your frappés using the Vaganova Method, where the foot is in sur le cou-de-pied on the ankle before it is extended (2.5.21), or the Cecchetti Method, where the foot is flexed at the ankle and pointed as it is extended. (2.5.22) You may also choose to do a combination of both.

155

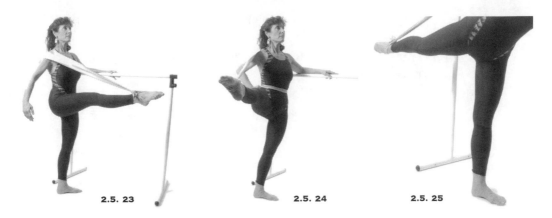

2.5. 23   2.5. 24   2.5. 25

7. DÉVELOPÉ

  a. Dévelopé the R leg from first position through retiré in any combination or at any height that your flexibility will permit.

  b. Repeat the combination en croix. (2.5.23, 2.5.24, and 2.5.25)

   • You may use your R hand to increase the tension as your leg extends in each direction.

  c. Turn around, change the band, and repeat a.–b. with the L leg.

8. GRAND BATTEMENT

  a. Grand battement the R leg en croix.

   • Make sure your body stays stable throughout the exercise.

   • Adjust the band tension if necessary.

  b. Turn around, change the band, and repeat with the L leg.

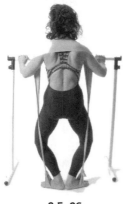
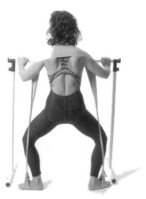

2.5. 26   2.5. 27

9. JUMPS AT THE BARRE

STARTING POSITION: Attach each end of the band under the sole of each foot. Spread the center of the band across your shoulders. Face the barre and hold the barre with both hands.

EXERCISE:

a. Work on your jumps.

- Small jumps in first (2.5.26) and second positions (2.5.27).
- Changement in fifth position.
- Bigger jumps.

Lessons from Life

#1. ALIGNMENT TAKES TIME

When dancers come to me before a performance with aches and pains, I usually will do just relaxation work with them, specifically avoiding any deep tissue work so as to not disturb their alignment. The alignment they are familiar with must remain their "comfort zone" until after show time—even if their present alignment is causing stress on the body and is the reason for their discomfort. Learning good alignment and correcting bad posture habits is a process that takes time and attention and is not something that can be "fixed" all at once.

#2. POWERFUL BACK

Once we sustain an injury, it may become necessary to find an alternative way to handle movement. This way the stress can be redistributed through the body, rather than just on the injured part. I had a college athlete who came to see me because the swimming scholarship he had was about to be reevaluated. He had a severe elbow injury which held back his swimming progress. I looked at his swimming movement and observed that he used primarily his arm and shoulder muscles, pushing through the pain, fighting his body to do what it was not yet ready to do. During our time together, I showed him how to initiate the swimming motion from his back muscles, which were strong and had not been injured. The arm would be able to carry the movement as a result, but the power would come from the back.

#3. TREAT THE WHOLE BODY

Occasionally, an injured student will come to me for a quick *miracle fix*. With young adults (especially dancers), I can get muscles to respond faster and let go of the tension sooner than with older people. However, even the youngest and most flexible bodies need more than instant "magic" to work with their injuries. It is important to treat the situation that caused the injury as well as the injury itself in order to prevent it from happening again. You may even find that it is necessary to completely relearn a movement pattern in another way, so that the same thing will not occur again. The injured area must be healed and strengthened. Look at your alignment in a functional way by asking yourself, "How can I move using the correct muscles to create balance and harmony?"

Conclusion

Conclusion

As you have read and experimented with these exercises, I hope you have been able to take on an attitude and mind-set of *awareness*, which I have tried to convey to you.

I am sure that by now you recognize some of the following benefits of using the Thera-Band® as you warm up and workout. Thera-Bands® . . .

1. provide the appropriate resistance in order to increase the strength and flexibility of the muscles;
2. allow movement in three dimensions;
3. make initiating movement from the pelvis easier to achieve;
4. integrate different body parts to achieve harmonious and fluent movement;
5. get in touch with the capacities of the spine for extension, flexion, and rotation, and for recognizing the relationship between the head and the tailbone;
6. provide support and balance, in some exercises;
7. allow full range of movement (for example, using the complete range of capabilities of the hip when turning);
8. provide a reference for posture and alignment that will reflect on your everyday activities; and,
9. provide the tactile sensation on the skin, thus provoking greater awareness.

I hope you will continue to work with the Thera-Band®, using your own knowledge and creativity to develop other exercises that are specifically suited to meeting the needs of your own individual body.

Bibliography

Bibliography

Alexander, F. Matthias. *The Alexander Technique: The Essential Writings of F. Matthias Alexander*. Selected and introduced by Edward Maisel. London: Thames and Hudson, 1990.

———. *The Use of the Self*. New York: E. P. Dutton & Co., 1932. Reprint. Long Beach, CA: Centerline Press, 1984.

Alexander, Gerda. *Eutony: The Holistic Discovery of the Total Person*. New York: Felix Morrow, 1985.

Alter, Michael J. *Science of Stretching*. Champaign, IL: Human Kinetics Books, 1988.

———. *Sport Stretch*. Champaign, IL: Leisure Press, 1990.

Brooks, Charles V.W. *Sensory Awareness: The Rediscovery of Experiencing Through Workshops With Charlotte Selver*. New York: Viking Press, 1974. Reprint. New York: Felix Morrow, 1986.

Chmelar, Robin D. and Sally S. Fitt. *Dancing at Your Peak: Diet: A Complete Guide To Nutrition and Weight Control*. Pennington, NJ: Princeton Book Company, 1990.

Clarkson, Priscilla M. and Margaret Skrinar, eds. *Science of Dance Training*. Champaign, IL: Human Kinetics Books, 1988.

Clarkson, Priscilla, Oded Bar-Or, and David R. Lamb. *Exercise and the Female: A Life Span Approach. Perspectives in Exercise Science and Sports Medicine*, vol. 9. Carmel, IN: Cooper Publishing Group, 1996.

Cohen, Bonnie Bainbridge. "The Action in Perceiving," *Contact Quarterly*, 12, no. 3 (Fall 1987): 22–26.

———. "The Dancer's Warm-up through Body-Mind Centering." *Contact Quarterly*, 13, no. 3 (Fall 1988): 28–29.

———. "Perceiving in Action," *Contact Quarterly*, 9, no. 2 (Spring/Summer 1984): 24–39.

———. "Relationship of the Concept of Proximal and Distal Initiation to Muscle Structure and Function." Amherst, MA: The School for Body/Mind Centering, 1977.

———. *Sensing, Feeling, and Action: The Experiential Anatomy of Body-Mind Centering: The Collected Articles from Contact Quarterly Dance Journal, 1980–1992*. Northampton, MA: Contact Editions, 1993.

Dowd, Irene. *Taking Root to Fly: Ten Articles on Functional Anatomy*. New York: Contact Collaborations, Inc., 1981. 3rd rev. ed. New York: Irene Dowd, 1995.

Feldenkrais, Moshe. *Awareness Through Movement: Health Exercises for Personal Growth*. New York: Harper & Row, Publishers, Inc., 1972. Reprint. New York: HarperCollins, 1990.

———. *The Elusive Obvious*. Cupertino, CA: Meta Publications, 1981.

———. *The Potent Self: A Guide to Spontaneity*. New York: Harper & Row, Publishers, Inc., 1985. Reprint. San Francisco: HarperSanFrancisco, 1992.

Fitt, Salley Sevey. *Dance Kinesiology 2nd edition*. New York: Schirmer Books, 1996.

Friden, J. "Changes in Human Skeletal Muscle Induced by Long-Term Eccentric Exercise." *Cell Tissue Research*, 236, no. 2 (1984): 365–372.

Friden, J., Sjostrom, M., and B. Ekblom. *Experimentia* 37, no. 5 (1981): 506–507.

Grant, Gail. *Technical Manual and Dictionary of Classical Ballet*, third revised edition. New York: Dover Publications, Inc., 1982.

Hoppenfeld, Stanley and Richard Hutton. *Physical Examination of the Spine and Extremities*. Norwalk, CT: Appleton-Century-Crofts, 1976.

Hygienic Corporation. *Thera-Band® System of Progressive Resistance: Instruction Manual, vol. 3*. OH: The Hygienic Corporation, 1992.

Juhan, Deane. *Job's Body: A Handbook for Bodywork*. Barringtown, New York: Station Hill Press/Barrytown, 1987. Expanded edition. Barrington, NY: Barrytown, Ltd, 1998.

Kapit, Wynn and Lawrence M. Elson. *The Anatomy Coloring Book*. New York: Harper Collins Publishers, Inc., 1977. Second edition. New York: Addison Wesley Publishing Company: 1993.

Kedall, Florence Peterson and Elizabeth Kendall McCreary. *Muscles: Testing and Function, Fourth edition*. Baltimore: Lippincott, Williams & Wilkins, 1993.

Kirstein, Lincoln and Muriel Stuart. *The Classical Ballet: Basic Technique and Terminology*. New York: Alfred A. Knopf, Inc., 1952. Reprint. Gainsville: University Press of Florida, 1998.

Lao Tzu. *Tao Te Ching*. Translated by Victor H. Mair. New York: Quality Paperback Book Club, 1990.

Linden, Paul. *Compute in Comfort*. Saddle River, NJ: Prentice-Hall, Inc., 1995.

———. "Being in Movement: Intention as a Somatic Meditation," *Somatics*, (Autumn/Winter 1988–89): 54–59.

McMinn, R. M. H. and R. T. Hutchings. *A Color Atlas of Human Anatomy*. London: Wolfe Medical Publications Ltd., 1977.

Mariechild, Diane. *The Inner Dance*. Freedom, CA: The Crossing Press, 1987.

Marks, S. C., R. M. H. McMinn, Peter H. Abrahams, and Ralph T. Hutchings. *McMinn's Color Atlas of Human Anatomy, Fourth Edition*. London: Mosby-Year Book, 1998.

McAtee, Robert E. *Facilitated Stretching*. Colorado Springs, CO: Human Kinetics Publishers, 1993.

Minton, Sandra Cerny. *Body and Self: Partners in Movement*. Champaign, IL: Human Kinetics Publishers, 1989.

Morris, Christopher M. *The Complete Guide to Stretching*. London: A. & C. Black, Ltd., 1999.

Nelson, Lisa, and Nancy Stark Smith. "Interview with Bonnie Bainbridge Cohen." *Contact Quarterly* 5, no. 2 (Winter 1980): 20–28.

Newham, D. J., G. McPhail, K. R. Mills, & R. H. T. Edwards. "Ultra Structural Changes After Concentric and Eccentric Contraction of Human Muscle." *Journal of the Neurological Sciences*, 61, no. 1 (1983): 109–122.

Olsen, Andrea, in collaboration with Caryn McHose. *BodyStories: A Guide to Experimental Anatomy*. Barrytown, NY: Station Hill Press, Inc., 1991. Expanded edition. Barrytown, NY: Station Hill Ltd., 1999.

Rolf, Ida, Ph.D. *Rolfing: The Integration of Human Structure*. New York: Harper & Row, Publishers, 1977.

Saltonstall, Ellen. *Kinetic Awareness: Discovering Your Bodymind*. New York: Kinetic Awareness Center, 1988.

School for Body/Mind Centering. *Ontogenetic and Phylogenetic Developmental Principles, revised edition*. Amherst, MA: School for Body/Mind Centering, 1977.

———. *Organs: Lungs, Heart, Kidneys, Bladder, Gonads, revised edition*. Amherst, MA: School for Body/Mind Centering, 1977.

———. *Skeletal System, revised edition*. Amherst, MA: School for Body/Mind Centering, 1977.

Selim, Robert D. *Muscles: The Magic of Motion: The Human Body*. Human Body Series. Washington, D.C.: U.S. News & World Report, Inc., 1982.

Smith, Fritz Frederick. *Inner Bridges: A Guide to Energy Movement and Body Structure*. Atlanta, GA: Humanics Publishing Group, 1986.

Smith, Nancy Stark. "Living Anatomy of Vision: Interview With Bonnie Bainbridge Cohen." *Contact Quarterly*, 6: no. 1 (Winter 1981): 5–9.

Spector-Flock, Noa. "The Power of Stretching with a Band." Unpublished article, 2001.

Syer, John and Christopher Connolly. *Sporting Body, Sporting Mind: An Athlete's Guide to Mental Training*. Englewood, NJ: Prentice-Hall, Inc., 1989.

Thomasen, Eivind and Rachel-Anne Rist. *Anatomy and Kinesiology for Ballet Teachers*. London: Dance Books, 1996.

Thompson, Clem W. *Manual of Structural Kinesiology, 11th edition*. St. Louis, MO: Times Mirror/Mosby College Publishing, 1989.

Thoreau, Henry David. *Walden and Other Writings*. New York: Barnes and Noble, 1993.

Travell, Janet G. and David G. Simons. *Myofascial Pain and Dysfunction: The Trigger Point Manual. 2 vols. Second Edition*. Baltimore: Lippincott, Williams & Wilkins, 1998.

Watkins, Andrea and Priscilla M. Clarkson. *Dancing Longer, Dancing Stronger: A Dancer's Guide to Improving Technique and Preventing Injury*. Pennington, NJ: Princeton Book Company, 1990.

Appendix A
General Terms

1. **abductors:** any muscle group that will bring a particular body part away from the midline of the body (e.g., raising the arm out to the side). (A.1)

2. **adductors:** any muscle group that will bring a particular body part closer to the body's midline (e.g., when sitting on a chair and crossing one leg over the other, the inner thigh muscle will adduct the leg over the other leg.) (A.2)

3. **anterior:** the front of the body or specific body part. (A.3)

4. **circumduction:** the moving of a bone in a circular pattern from a single pivot point, creating a cone shape in space. (A.4)

5. **concentric:** when the distance between muscle ends becomes shorter in a contraction. (See page 22 for more information.) (A.5)

6. **contraction:** the building of tension in a muscle or muscle group. The muscle fibers may shorten (concentric contraction), lengthen (eccentric contraction), or stay the same (isometric contraction).

7. **depression:** the downward motion of a body part, or the returning movement from elevation.

8. **dorsal:** the upper side of a body part.

9. **eccentric:** when muscle fibers become more extended and the distance between the two muscle ends is greater in a contraction. (See page 22 for more information.) (A.6)

10. **elevation:** the upward motion of a body part.

11. eversion: the outward rotation of the foot from the midline of the body. (A.7)

12. extension: straightening; moving bones apart to make the angle between them wider. (A.8)

A.7

13. fixation: the stabilizing or fixating of one area of the body while another area moves freely.

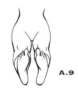

A.8

14. flexed foot: the bringing of the top (dorsal side) of the foot and all toes toward the front part of the leg. (A.9)

A.9

15. flexion: the bending of a joint where the angle between two bones becomes smaller.

16. frontal plane: a division of the body that creates separate back and front regions. (A.10)

17. horizontal extension (abduction): the movement of a body part in the horizontal plane backward from the front of the body to the side (e.g., moving the lifted arm from in front of the chest to the side).

18. horizontal flexion (adduction): movement of a body part horizontally from the side of the body to the front (e.g., moving the lifted arm from the side of the body to in front of the chest).

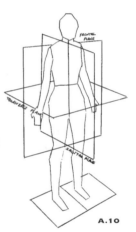

A.10

19. horizontal plane (also called transverse plane): a division of the body at the waistline that creates an upper region and a lower region of the body. (A.10)

20. hyperextension: when a joint (especially the knee and elbow joints) that is designed to flex in only one direction is straightened to a locked position, sometimes to the point that it begins to flex in the opposite direction.

21. inversion: the turning inward of the foot, for example, so the sole is facing toward the midline of the body. (A.11)

22. ischial tuberosity: one of the two "sitting bones"; the lowest of the three protruding bones of the pelvis (the others being the illium and the pubis). (A.12)

A.11

ISCHIAL TUBEROSITIES

A.12

23. **lateral:** the side or outer aspect of the body or a body part.

24. **lumbar region:** the five vertebras located between the mid-back and the top of the hip (pelvis) at the waistline. (A.13)

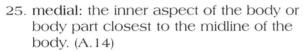
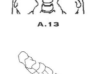

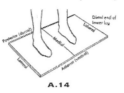
A.13

25. **medial:** the inner aspect of the body or body part closest to the midline of the body. (A.14)

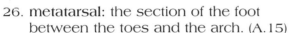
A.14

26. **metatarsal:** the section of the foot between the toes and the arch. (A.15)

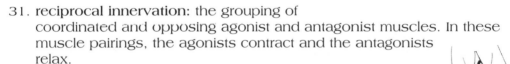
A.15

27. **plantar:** the lower side or aspect of a body part, for example, the sole of the foot.

28. **pointed foot:** the plantar flexion of the foot where the foot is extended to be in line with the lower part of the leg. (A.16)

A.16

29. **posterior:** the back side of the body.

30. **prone position:** lying on your abdomen, face down. (A.17)

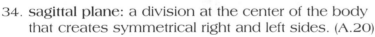
A.17

31. **reciprocal innervation:** the grouping of coordinated and opposing agonist and antagonist muscles. In these muscle pairings, the agonists contract and the antagonists relax.

32. **rotation:** the moving of a bone along its own axis. (A.18)

33. **sacrum:** the flat, triangular-shaped bone located on the back (posterior aspect) of the pelvis, at the end of the lumbar area and between the two hipbones (iliac crests). (A.19)

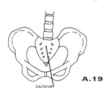
A.18

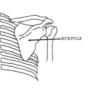
A.19

34. **sagittal plane:** a division at the center of the body that creates symmetrical right and left sides. (A.20)

35. **scapula:** the shoulder blade, which is a triangular-shaped, somewhat flat bone. (A.21)

A.21

36. **sickled foot:** the disruption of good foot alignment caused by turning the toes inward, as if you were looking at the sole of your foot. (A.22)

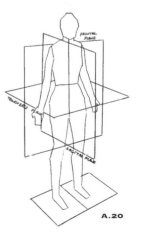

A.22

A.20

37. **subluxation:** partial dislocation. An example may be a hip that "snaps" on leg flexion, even getting out of the socket. It represents the loss of joint integrity, but the bones do return to normal.

38. **supine position:** lying on your back, face up. (A.23)

A.23

Appendix B
Ballet Terms, Russian Style

1. **à la seconde**: a positioning of the arms or the legs directly to the side of the body, as if in a second position. (B.1)

2. **arabesque**: a body position in which one leg is extended directly behind you, often at a 90° angle from the standing leg. You are supported on the other leg, which may be bent or straight. Several arm positions can be used to create a long line from the toes to the fingers. Both shoulders are equal, as well as both hips, and both are at right angles to the line of direction. (B.2)

3. **attitude**: a body position in which you are standing on one leg with the other leg bent at a 90° angle from thigh to lower leg. The lifted leg is either directly front (devant), side (à la seconde), or behind (derrière). (B.3)

4. **changement**: a jump straight up in the air during which the legs switch from a fifth position with one foot in front to land in a fifth position with the other foot in front. (B.4)

5. **derrière**: a movement or stationary position that involves moving a limb directly behind the body or moving the whole body toward the back.

6. **devant**: a stationary position or movement that involves moving a limb directly in front of the body or moving the whole body toward the front.

7. **développé**: a stationary movement that is done while standing on one leg. The thigh of the other leg is lifted, with the toes of the lifted leg touching the standing leg as they are drawn up. (B.5) As soon as the thigh reaches maximum height, it is held there while the lower leg

B.1

B.2

B.3

B.4

leaves the standing leg and is fully extended to a straight position in the air as in arabesque. (B.6)

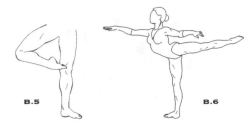

B.5   B.6

8. **en croix:** literally, "in the shape of a cross"; working in all directions—to the front, side, back, and side of the body again.

9. **plié:** a bend of the knees while standing. It can be **demi-plié** (half bend), in which the torso goes as low as possible when the knees bend and the heels do not lift off the floor, or it can be **grand plié** (large bend), a deep bend of the knees in which the heels do come off the floor (except in second position).

10. **relevé (half toe):** standing on one or both feet, lift the heels off the floor so your weight moves to the balls of your feet. (B.7)

B.7

11. **retiré:** literally "withdrawn"; a position in which the thigh is lifted with the toe at the supporting leg's knee. (B.5)

12. **rond de jambe:** a circular movement of the leg. It can be done with the toes remaining on the floor (à terre) or with the leg lifted in the air (en l'air), and the circle can be outward (**en dehors,** away from the standing leg) or inward (**en dedans,** toward the working leg).

13. **sauté:** a jump straight up in the air. The position on the ground is the same before the jump and after it; it does not change in the air.

14. **sur le cou-de-pied:** a stationary position with the sole of one foot wrapped around the ankle of the standing foot, so that the heel can be seen from the front and the toes are behind the Achilles tendon of the standing foot. (B.8)

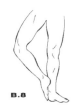

B.8

15. **tendu:** a stationary movement standing on one leg. The other foot slides out in a particular direction (the knee is straight) and the toes remain on the floor. (B.9)

B.9

16. **turn-in:** the inward rotation of the legs in the hip sockets.

17. **turn-out:** the outward rotation of the legs in the hip sockets, very important and basic to all ballet movements and positions. (B.10)

B.10

Appendix C
Positions of the Feet, Legs, Body, and Arms

1. **all-fours position:** body weight is on the hands and knees, with the thighs and the arms at a 90° angle to the torso. (C.1)

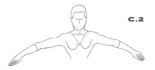

C.1

2. **ballet positions of the arms, Russian style:**

   A. **first position:** arms are held out in front of the body in a circular position, so that the hands are at about the height of your navel, elbows are slightly bent and facing outward, tips of the fingers are almost touching, and palms are facing toward your body.

   B. **second position:** arms are in the same shape as first position, except they are held out to each side of the body. (C.2)

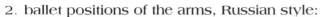

C.2

   C. **third position:** arms are in the same shape as first position, except both arms are lifted so the hands are above the head with fingers almost touching. This corresponds to the Cecchetti fifth position en haut and the French School's fifth position.

3. **ballet positions of the feet:**

   A. **first position:** heels are together, legs are turned out at the hip socket so the toes and knees point out from each other on a diagonal, as far as the hip socket allows. (C.3)

C.3

   B. **second position:** same as first position, except feet are about hips-width apart or wider. (C.4)

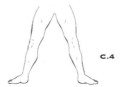

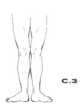

C.4

C. third position: similar to first position, except the heel of one foot is touching the instep of the other foot. This position is rarely used. (C.5)

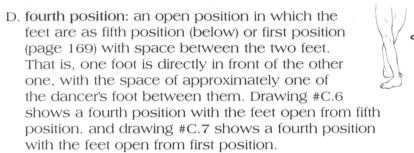

C.5

D. fourth position: an open position in which the feet are as fifth position (below) or first position (page 169) with space between the two feet. That is, one foot is directly in front of the other one, with the space of approximately one of the dancer's foot between them. Drawing #C.6 shows a fourth position with the feet open from fifth position. and drawing #C.7 shows a fourth position with the feet open from first position.

C.6

C.7

E. fifth position: legs are rotated outward at the hip; one foot is in front of the other, so that the outside edge (lateral aspect) of the heel of the front foot is touching the big toe of the back foot. (Ideally, the outside edge of the little toe of the front foot is touching the medial aspect of the heel of the back foot as well.) (C.8)

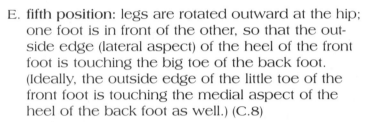

C.8

C.9

4. sitting fourth position: sitting on the floor, one leg is bent in a 90° angle in front of the body, turned outward, and the other leg is bent in a 90° angle behind the body, turned inward; this creates an open square shape with the legs. (C.9)

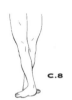

5. sitting parallel first position: sitting on the floor, legs are directly forward, the legs are in front of the hip joints, knees straight and directed toward the ceiling (i.e., not turned out). (C.10)

C.10

6. sitting wide second position: sitting on the floor: straddle split; legs are open wide to each side of the body, knees straightened and directed toward the ceiling (i.e., not turned out). (C.11)

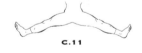

C.11

7. standing parallel first position: feet are parallel to each other (i.e., not turned out) a few inches apart. (C.12)

8. standing parallel second position: feet are parallel to each other (i.e., not turned out), about hips-width apart (i.e. using the outside of the pelvis as the measure). (C.13)

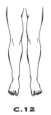

C.12

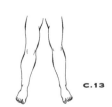

C.13

Appendix D
Three-Part Whole Body Program (Sample)

I. FIRST DAY

1. Abdominals: The Ice Cream Scooper (Pg. 43)
2. Abdominals: Rotation (Pg. 45)
3. Iliopsoas Stretch (Pg. 48)
4. Leg Stretch (Pg. 49)
5. Spinal Chain (Pg. 51)
6. Antigravity Leg Work (#1–4) (Pg. 61)
7. Lying on One Side (#1–9) (Pg. 67)
8. The Hinge (Pg. 73)
9. The Little Mermaid's Tail (Pg. 79)
10. The Pendulum (Pg. 83)
11. The Body Builder (#1 only) (Pg. 131)
12. Prone: The Archer's Bow (Pg. 133)
13. Deep Rotation of the Back (Pg. 135)
14. Antigravity Foot Work (Pg. 85)
15. Pearl Necklace (#1) (Pg. 138)

I. ALTERNATING DAY

1. Abdominals: The Ice Cream Scooper (Pg. 43)
2. Abdominals: Rotation (Pg. 45)
3. Iliopsoas Stretch (Pg. 48)
4. Leg Stretch (Pg. 49)
5. Spinal Chain (Pg. 51)
6. The Traffic Director (#1–6) (Pg. 107)
7. The Chest Press (Pg. 99)
8. The Shawl (Pg. 100)
9. The Crescent Bend (Pg. 102)
10. Laterals (Pg. 128)
11. The Body Builder (Pg. 131)
12. Prone: The Archer's Bow (#2 only) (Pg. 135)
13. Pearl Necklace (#3) (Pg. 138)

II. FIRST DAY

1. Abdominals: The Ice Cream Scooper (Pg. 43)
2. Abdominals: Rotation (Pg. 45)
3. Abdominal Combination (Pg. 46)
4. Iliopsoas Stretch (Pg. 48)
5. Spinal Chain (Pg. 51)
6. Antigravity Leg Work (Pg. 61)
7. The Stork Leg Work (Pg. 88)
8. Lying on One Side (#1–6 and 10–13) (Pg. 67)
9. Posterior: The Jungle Cat (#1–3 and #5–9) (Pg. 74)
10. Leg Adductors (Pg. 84)
11. P.N.F.: The Infinity Symbol (Pg. 125)
12. The Body Builder (Pg. 131)
13. The Archer's Bow (Pg. 133)
14. Deep Rotation of the Back (Pg. 135)

II. ALTERNATING DAY

1. Abdominals: The Ice Cream Scooper (Pg. 43)
2. Abdominals: Rotation (Pg. 45)
3. Abdominal Combination (Pg. 46)
4. Iliopsoas Stretch (Pg. 48)
5. Spinal Chain (Pg. 51)
6. The Traffic Director (#1–5 and #7–9) (Pg. 107)
7. Biceps (Pg. 105)
8. Triceps (Pg. 106)
9. The Crescent Bend (Pg. 102)
10. Hands of the Clock (Pg. 104)
11. The Body Builder (Pg. 131)
12. The Archer's Bow (#2 only) (Pg. 133)
13. Pearl Necklace (#3–4) (Pg. 138)

III. FIRST DAY

1. Abdominals: The Ice Cream Scooper (Pg. 43)
2. Abdominals: Rotation (Pg. 45)
3. Abdominal Combination (Pg. 46)
4. Iliopsoas Stretch (Pg. 48)
5. Spinal Chain (Pg. 51)
6. The Traffic Director (#2–4 and #7–9) (Pg. 107)
7. Chest Press (Pg. 99)
8. The Shawl (Pg. 100)
9. The Crescent Bend (Pg. 102)
10. Half-Moon Twist (Pg. 127)
11. Laterals (Pg. 128)
12. The Body Builder (All) (Pg. 131)
13. Pearl Necklace (Pg. 138)

III. ALTERNATING DAY

1. Abdominals: The Ice Cream Scooper (Pg. 43)
2. Abdominals: Rotation (Pg. 45)
3. Abdominal Combination (Pg. 46)
4. Iliopsoas Stretch (Pg. 48)
5. Spinal Chain (Pg. 51)
6. Antigravity Leg Work (Pg. 61)
7. Posterior: The Jungle Cat (Pg. 74)
8. Strengthening the Adductors (Pg. 81)
9. Calf and Foot: Revving the Accelerator (Pg. 86)
10. Antigravity Foot Work (Pg. 85)
11. Working with a Barre (Pg. 140)
12. Preparation for Allegro Work (Pg. 151)

Appendix E
Program for Dance Conditioning

(SAMPLE) FIRST DAY

1. Abdominals: The Ice Cream Scooper (Pg. 43)
2. Abdominals: Rotation (Pg. 45)
3. Abdominal Combination (Pg. 46)
4. Iliopsoas Stretch (Pg. 48)
5. Spinal Chain (Pg. 51)
6. Leg Stretch (Pg. 49)
7. Antigravity Leg Work (Pg. 61)
8. Advanced Antigravity Leg Work (Pg. 66)
9. The Stork Leg Work (for plié, balance, extension) (Pg. 88)
10. Lying on One Side (#1–7; for passé, retiré, and extension) (Pg. 67)
11. The Hinge, Hamstring Stretch (Pg. 73)
12. Posterior: The Jungle Cat (#3, 4, 7–9) (Pg. 74)
13. The Little Mermaid's Tail (Pg. 79)
14. The Pendulum (Pg. 83)
15. Leg Adductors (Pg. 84)
16. Antigravity Foot Work (Pg. 85)
17. Calf and Foot: Revving the Accelerator (Pg. 86)
18. The Body Builder (Pg. 131)
19. The Archer's Bow (Pg. 133)
20. Deep Rotation of the Back (Pg. 135)
21. Deep Rotation of the Upper Torso (Pg. 137)
22. Pearl Necklace (Pg. 138)

ALTERNATING DAY

1. Abdominals: The Ice Cream Scooper (Pg. 43)
2. Abdominals: Rotation (Pg. 45)
3. Abdominal Combination (Pg. 46)
4. Iliopsoas Stretch (Pg. 48)
5. Spinal Chain (Pg. 51)
6. The Traffic Director (#1–4) (Pg. 107)
7. The Shawl (Pg. 100)
8. Chest Press (Pg. 99)
9. Crescent Bend (Pg. 102)
10. Half-moon Twist (Pg. 127)
11. Laterals (Pg. 128)
12. The Body Builder (Pg. 131)
13. The Archer's Bow (Pg. 133)
14. Deep Rotation of the Back (Pg. 135)
15. Deep Rotation of the Upper Torso (Pg. 137)
16. Pearl Necklace (Pg. 138)

Appendix F
Program for Swim Conditioning

(SAMPLE) FIRST DAY

1. Abdominals: The Ice Cream Scooper (Pg. 43)
2. Abdominals: Rotation (Pg. 45)
3. Abdominal Combination (for the warm-up of the back) (Pg. 46)
4. Iliopsoas Stretch (Pg. 48)
5. Lying on One Side (#1–3 to learn hip separation; #4 to strengthen the tensor fasciae latae) (Pg. 67)
6. The Hinge (Pg. 73)
7. The Little Mermaid's Tail (for posterior hip muscle) (Pg. 79)
8. Leg Adductors (for breast-stroke) (Pg. 84)
9. P.N.F.: The Infinity Symbol: ∞) (for overall coordination of leg and hip) (Pg. 125)
10. The Archer's Bow (Pg. 133)
11. Deep Rotation of the Back (Pg. 135)
12. Deep Rotation of the Upper Torso (Pg. 137)
13. Antigravity Foot Work (Pg. 85)
14. Calf and Foot: Revving the Accelerator (Pg. 86)

ALTERNATING DAY

1. Abdominals: The Ice Cream Scooper (Pg. 43)
2. Abdominals: Rotation (Pg. 45)
3. Abdominal Combination (Pg. 46)
4. Iliopsoas Stretch (Pg. 48)
5. Lying on One Side (#1–4) (Pg. 67)
6. The Hinge (Pg. 73)
7. P.N.F.: Infinity Symbol: ∞ (Pg. 125)
8. The Traffic Director (Pg. 107)
9. Chest Press (Pg. 99)
10. Biceps (Pg. 105)
11. Triceps (Pg. 106)
12. The Shawl (Pg. 100)
13. The Crescent Bend (for the side rib muscles) (Pg. 102)
14. The Body Builder (Pg. 131)

Where can I buy Thera-Band®?

Thera-Band® is available either through local medical supply stores, the internet, or author Noa Spector-Flock.

THROUGH THERA-BAND® DEALERS:

Thera-Band® is manufactured by The Hygenic Corporation. You can contact the company directly to find a dealer near you. The following information is accurate as of 2001. Updated information is always on the company's website, <www.thera-band.com>.

In the United States or Canada:
1-800-321-2135
Monday–Friday: 8 a.m.–5 p.m. ET
The Hygenic Corporation
1245 Home Avenue
Akron, Ohio 44310

Outside the United States:
330-633-8460
330-633-9359 (fax)
Thera-Band GmbH Mainzer
Landstrasse 19
D-65589 Hadamar, Germany
+49 6433 91640;
+49 6433 9164 (fax)

THROUGH THE INTERNET:

Fitness Wholesale is a large distributor for Thera-Band®. Their web address for Thera-Band® is <www.fwonline.com/tbands.htm>

An Internet search using the keyword "Thera-Band" will list several other websites offering sales of Thera-Bands®.

FROM THE AUTHOR:

You may also purchase Thera-Band® directly from Noa Spector-Flock, through her e-mail address, <noanik8@att.net> or by telephone at 1-727-345-2570.

Get
STRONGER
by
STRETCHING
with Thera-Band®

is accompanied by a three-video set, now available from Dance Horizons Videos

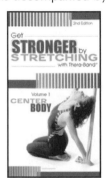

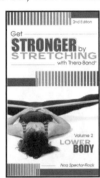

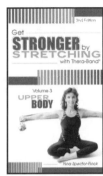

Volume I: Center of Body
50 minutes, color, 2001
$30.00

Volume II: Lower Body
63 minutes, color, 2001
$30.00

Volume III: Upper Body
31 minutes, color, 2001
$20.00

Noa Spector-Flock's exercise program helps you look, feel and move better. Using the Thera-Band® enhances output by making the most of your time and energy. The workout creates flexibility supported by strength, coordination, increased circulation, and graceful movement. The videos include lying down, sitting and standing exercises. Spector-Flock gives clear verbal directions and easy-to-follow demonstrations for each exercise. Each video includes information for purchasing your Thera-Band®.

GET **STRONGER** BY **STRETCHING** with Thera-Band® *Video Order Form*

Name _____ Phone _____

Address _____

City _____ State _____ Zip _____

PAYMENT OPTIONS

❏Check $ _____ ❏ VISA ❏M/C ❏AMEX

Account # _____

Signature _____

Mail to:
Princeton Book Company, Publishers,
PO Box 831, Hightstown, NJ 08520
Order by phone: 609-426-0602 or 800-220-7149 (US only)
Mon-Fri, 9-5 e.s.t.
Order by fax: 609-426-1344
Order by e-mail: pbc@dancehorizons.com

Please allow 1-2 weeks for delivery. Shipments to US addresses are sent by UPS or Priority Mail. Please add $5 for the first title, $2 for each additional title. Shipments outside the US must be paid by credit card. Shipping and handling charges will depend on the weight of your purchase and its destination.

Please send me these
"Get **Stronger** by **Stretching**
with Thera-Band®" *videos*

Quantity ❏ **Volume I: Center of Body**		$30.00
Quantity ❏ **Volume II: Lower Body**		$30.00
Quantity ❏ **Volume III: Upper Body**		$20.00
Subtotal		_____
Shipping and handling fee		_____
NJ residents, add 6% sales tax		_____
Total payment enclosed		_____